GRAVE DEALINGS

Body Snatching in Philadelphia, 1762–1883

TIM DEWYSOCKIE

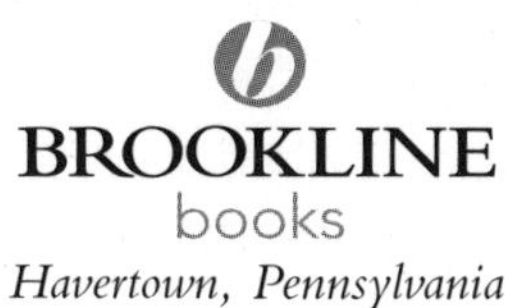

Havertown, Pennsylvania

Brookline Books is an imprint of Casemate Publishers

Published in the United States of America and Great Britain in 2025 by
BROOKLINE BOOKS
1950 Lawrence Road, Havertown, PA 19083, USA
and
47 Church Street, Barnsley, S70 2AS, UK

Paperback Edition: ISBN 978-1-955041-12-6
Digital Edition: ISBN 978-1-955041-13-3

A CIP record for this book is available from the British Library

Printed and bound in the United Kingdom by CPI Group (UK) Ltd, Croydon, CR0 4YY
Typeset in India by DiTech Publishing Services

For a complete list of Brookline Books titles, please contact:

CASEMATE PUBLISHERS (US)
Telephone (610) 853-9131
Fax (610) 853-9146
Email: casemate@casematepublishers.com
www.casematepublishers.com

CASEMATE PUBLISHERS (UK)
Telephone (0)1226 734350
Email: casemate@casemateuk.com
www.casemateuk.com

Cover image: "A Resurrectionist in Albany nearly buried alive by the caving in of the earth," March 26, 1859. (*Frank Leslie's Illustrated Newspaper*)

The Publisher's authorised representative in the EU for product safety is Authorised Rep Compliance Ltd., Ground Floor, 71 Lower Baggot Street, Dublin D02 P593, Ireland.
www.arccompliance.com

Contents

Acknowledgements

This book is based on research conducted for my master's thesis "Body Snatching in Philadelphia: A Social and Cultural History, 1762–1883," which was written with the invaluable, generous feedback of my advisor Dr. Joy Wiltenburg during the COVID-19 pandemic. I also want to thank Dr. William Carrigan and Dr. Janet Lindman for their input as part of my thesis committee, as well as all the history faculty I had the pleasure of taking courses with at Rowan University. This book would not have been possible without their direction.

I want to thank Angelina Brown and Lauren Gibbs for introducing me to body snatching when I was searching for a topic to write about for my class on the History of Crime, which led to this book. Rowan University's Campbell Library Access Services department was invaluable to securing the sources needed for writing this book through the magic of interlibrary loan: Daniel Pugh, Abigail Hummell-Bell, Melinda Ballard, Dylan Bieber, Shelby Brown, Laura Daniels, Nancy Demaris, Chante Dingle, Judith Kinkade, Jasmine Larzelere, Caitlin Packard-Howey, and Matthew Rosser. I am also indebted to many archives and other individuals. I want to thank Thomas Jefferson University's University Archivist and Head of Historic Collections F. Michael Angelo for guiding me through the institution's holdings on Philadelphia's 1882 body-snatching scandal.

Thanks to the Massachusetts Historical Society for providing copies of letters that were essential to this book, to the Library of Congress for, in the course of writing this book, digitizing other letters that were equally crucial, the Arlington Cemetery Company for putting me in touch with the owner of the Museum of Mourning Art's grave gun, and the Indiana

Archives and Records Administration for providing images and records of the Indianapolis body-snatcher Rufus Cantrell. Thanks also to Jennifer Green, Brookline Books, and Casemate for answering any and all of my questions in the process of writing and publishing this book. And of course, many thanks to Elayna, Gia, and my family for tolerating all the macabre finds I shared with them while writing this book.

GRAVE DEALINGS

Introduction

Death, Disinterment, and Dissection in Philadelphia

Her body dissected by fiendish man,
Her bones anatomized,
Her soul, we trust, has risen to God,
Where few physicians rise.

—RUTH SPRAGUE'S TOMBSTONE, NEAR HOOSICK FALLS, NEW YORK.
DIED JUNE 11, 1846, AGED NINE[1]

On a dark, frigid December night in 1882, a wagon came to a halt at Lebanon Cemetery in South Philadelphia. The driver waited while his two passengers entered a gap in the fence. A horrifying sight awaited the pair on the consecrated ground: six dead bodies. But they were not surprised. The cemetery's superintendent left them the "stiffs"—for three dollars apiece. They had a job to do, one they had done many times before. The men loaded the corpses into the wagon and departed for the local medical school, where students would dissect their macabre merchandise.[2]

Today we take for granted that when our loved ones are laid to rest, they will be at peace. Who would disturb them? But in 18th- and 19th-century America, burial grounds near medical schools suffered from a strange affliction: body snatching, the secret disinterment of the dead for medical education. Philadelphia—the birthplace of America, where the Declaration of Independence and Constitution were signed—was the site of many of the country's firsts, especially in medicine: the first hospital in 1751 (Pennsylvania Hospital), first anatomical lecture in 1762 (William Shippen Jr.), and the first medical school in 1765 (what would become the University of Pennsylvania). Shippen Jr. was also the first in the colonies to openly teach anatomy using human bodies. Following the model of European universities like Edinburgh where he was educated, Shippen's students learned to help the living by dismembering the dead.

Prominent 18th-century Scottish-born surgeon William Hunter wrote that dissection "informs the *head*, gives dexterity to the *hand*, and familiarizes the *heart* with a sort of necessary inhumanity [emphasis in original here and elsewhere in quoted matter]."[3] The gruesome reality of 18th- and 19th-century surgery called for a kind of "necessary inhumanity," or what today we would more politely call clinical detachment.[4] Before anesthesia, surgery was agonizing. According to historian Lindsey Fitzharris, the strength and speed of surgeons was prized as patients writhed in unimaginable pain; Robert Liston, a 19th-century British surgeon, could amputate a man's leg in under 30 seconds.[5] Dissection made surgeons more skillful, but it was also the primary method for understanding human anatomy, which led to more effective treatments and the advancement of medicine. The best anatomists were often the best surgeons, and taught both.[6]

But there was a problem: there were no volunteers who donated their bodies to science. Today fewer than 20,000 Americans, a fraction of 1 percent of the population, donate their bodies to medical schools annually, but it's still enough for students to be able to dissect their "first patient."[7] In the era of the body snatchers, that number was virtually zero. While it might seem obvious today that the best way to understand human anatomy is to study the human body, for much of history, social and religious opposition to dissection stymied progress.

Dissection was viewed literally as a fate worse than death: in 1752 it became a posthumous punishment for murder in Great Britain. The terror of dissection was so great that, facing the noose, some criminals were more afraid of being anatomized than executed. In 1788 a Boston highway robber wrote, "I was in a cold sweat; my knees smote together, and my tongue seemed to cleave to the roof of my mouth," at the prospect of his dissection, not his impending execution.[8] While intended to deter murder, the 1752 Murder Act also provided medical schools with a legal supply of corpses, a precedent followed in Philadelphia. But anatomists faced a dilemma. They needed more bodies for research and instruction than the legal system could provide, but there was only one other possible source: the dead interred in cemeteries. That is, if they were willing to take them, and violate the sanctity of the grave in the name of science. Philadelphia has a darker distinction, one that is not well known or understood: the birthplace of American medicine was also the birthplace of American body snatching.

The first body snatchers were physicians and their students, who made "most diligent use of the shovel and the scalpel" in the words of a New York medical student.[9] When Philadelphia pioneered American medicine and medical education in the 18th century, body snatching was small-scale and sporadic. But as the city became the center of the field in the following century, "professional" body snatchers emerged, middlemen who stole and sold corpses to the highest bidder. Anatomy was the cornerstone of the medical curriculum, and as medical schools proliferated, so did their need for anatomical "material." To paraphrase anthropologist Paul Wolff Mitchell, the price for Philadelphia's medical dominance was paid in cadavers.[10] What started as a crime of opportunity eventually became an underground market, with a size and scope that few were aware of at the time or even today. Bodies were even shipped across the country on trains in the "cadaver trade." Like other cities, secret agreements between city officials and medical schools sometimes regulated the plunder of public burial grounds in Philadelphia.

Those who trafficked in the dead went by many names. The general public referred to them as "grave robbers," the medical community as "resurrectionists," but they are best known today as "body snatchers."[11] They worked seasonally when medical schools were in session. Before modern embalming techniques, anatomy lectures were generally held in the colder months of the year to better preserve bodies for dissection. Body snatchers operated in the dead of night and approached graves on foot with the tools of their trade: a lantern to see, a shovel to dig, and a tool to pry coffins open.

Unearthing the entire grave was unnecessary. A hole was dug at the head of the coffin, deep and wide enough to clamber down and break it open, and an implement was placed around the body's neck to pull it out. Of course, it was quicker to remove corpses if cemetery staff were bribed to not bury them in the first place. While often called grave robbers, body snatchers were not interested in grave goods, and in fact were careful to leave everything behind *but* the body, such as clothing. Since human bodies could not be legally owned, body snatching was only a misdemeanor, but stealing clothing was a felony.[12] After evidence of the evening's incursion was hidden, bodies were usually transported by wagon to their destination. If they did the job right, mourners would leave flowers on empty graves, none the wiser.

Body snatching was profitable but also perilous. There was the possibility of jail time or fines, but punishment could be surprisingly light given how strongly people felt about the crime, especially when resurrectionists had powerful friends in the medical community. The real danger was vigilante justice, the wrath of communities. Colleges were ransacked in "anatomy riots." At night some burial grounds became battlegrounds, where traps were laid that, if triggered, would kill or maim unsuspecting body snatchers. Some believed the most appropriate punishment for body snatching was death. Advocates of cremation, a radical proposition in 1876 when the first American crematory was built in Pennsylvania, cited body snatching to support their arguments (today over half of Americans are cremated). It was a time when the dead needed protection from the living.

Body snatching produced such fierce resistance because, like dissection, it violated widely and deeply held beliefs and practices that dated back not just to the origins of Philadelphia, but all of human history. In 1681 King Charles II granted William Penn a charter to establish the colony that would become Pennsylvania. For the king of England it was a way to pay off his debt to Penn's father (an admiral in the Royal Navy who loaned the Crown 16,000 pounds). For Penn it was a way to create a "Holy Experiment," a refuge for Quakers like himself who rejected the Church of England, and members of other persecuted faiths, to freely practice their religion. The colony welcomed Jews, Anglicans, Mennonites, Lutherans, the African Methodist Episcopal Church, and other religious groups.[13] This toleration extended to beliefs about burial practices.

Quakers interred their dead according to the same principles they lived by: simply, unceremoniously, with plain gravestones, while other Protestant denominations used elaborate, decorative tombstones.[14] All Philadelphians memorialized their dead in meaningful ways, which was not surprising. As far back as archaeological records go, humans have always cared for the dead.[15]

What is surprising, and shocking, is when that care is denied. The denial of a "proper" burial, a fate reserved only for the most reviled in society, represents a denial of humanity. In England people who took their own lives were buried at crossroads with a stake driven through their heart, a practice that persisted until 1823 when it was outlawed by Parliament.[16] Similarly, body snatching and dissection were considered desecrations of the highest order, which was why some turned to violence in response. Body snatchers were referred to as "resurrectionists" because they performed their own twisted version of the Christian resurrection of the dead, at a time when it was widely believed that the body needed to remain whole in the grave for it to be later reunited with its soul in the afterlife.

Surprisingly little has been written about American body snatching, which might be because body snatching is most closely associated with cities like London and Edinburgh where it began. The most infamous case of body snatching in history, which wasn't really a case of body snatching at all, also occurred in Edinburgh, when the duo Burke and Hare murdered at least 16 people to sell their bodies to anatomists, a practice that would later be referred to as "burking." Ruth Richardson's *Death, Dissection, and the Destitute* analyzed Britain's 1832 Anatomy Act, which effectively ended body snatching in Great Britain, but resurrectionists continued to bedevil areas near American medical schools long after the practice ended in Europe.

Perhaps the most influential book on the subject is Michael Sappol's *A Traffic of Dead Bodies*, which focused primarily on body snatching in New York as part of a broader cultural history of anatomy. In *Body Snatching*, Suzanne M. Shultz provided a wide-ranging survey of the subject. Before these works and other significant studies, the history of body snatching was written from the perspective of the medical community.[17] In morally unproblematic narratives of medical progress, opposition to body snatching and dissection was chalked up to a "superstitious" public. Physicians of course presented themselves as the enlightened ones, even as many took steps to avoid being snatched and dissected themselves, such as delaying their burial until decomposition rendered it useless for study.

Philadelphia's medical preeminence came at a cost that was not borne equally. No one was truly safe, but body snatchers generally avoided so-called "respectable" burial grounds that, with greater resources, were better protected and drew more public scrutiny if body snatchers were caught there. Instead, they targeted the most vulnerable: Black cemeteries and public burial grounds where the poor, the unclaimed, and the unidentified were buried. Body snatchers pursued the path of least resistance, which usually meant victims fell along racial and class lines. But even that approach was not without risk, because Philadelphia's marginalized communities fought back against the medical community to defend their dead. Recent books like Daina Ramey Berry's *The Price for Their Pound of Flesh* explore understudied aspects of the history of body snatching, such as the links between the practice and slavery.

What's missing in the literature is a history of American body snatching in the city where it began: Philadelphia. Most focus on an infamous case of body snatching in 1882 that involved Jefferson Medical College (now part of Thomas Jefferson University), but that was the culmination of a much longer history. Because Philadelphia was so central to the practice, the history of body snatching in the city is really the history of body snatching in America.

This story also provides important context for understanding the present, because we are still living with the consequences of body snatching today. In 2024 the University of Pennsylvania's Penn Museum interred the skulls of 19 Black Philadelphians from its Morton Cranial Collection in Eden Cemetery. Named after Philadelphia doctor Samuel George Morton who collected them in the mid-19th century, the bones were used to support pseudoscience that linked skull structure to intelligence and gave a scientific veneer to the insidious beliefs underlying white supremacy and slavery.

The Mütter Museum, a Philadelphia medical history museum with a collection that includes slides of Einstein's brain, a "mega colon," and President Grover Cleveland's tumor, is conducting a review of its collection, while its *Postmortem Project* collects public feedback to shape the museum's future. There is a worldwide debate raging around the display and treatment of human remains. Is it ethical to display human remains, especially those obtained without consent, and who decides? In 2023 Harvard's morgue manager and others, including Pennsylvanians, were indicted in connection with the selling and buying of body parts in an interstate trade of human remains. While body snatchers of the past stole whole bodies for medical education, modern-day body snatchers exchange body parts in the "oddities" trade to build macabre personal collections.

Given the secretive nature of body snatching, its history is, so to speak, buried in the historical record. The grave dealings in these pages, unearthed from archives, newspapers, medical journals, and other sources, reveal a wide-ranging story that touches on the history of crime, cemeteries, and medical care. It begins in the 18th century when William Shippen Jr., the first professor of anatomy for America's first medical school, set off a firestorm in Philadelphia—including graveyard patrols and shootouts—by taking bodies from a public burial ground. Chapter 2 explores the troubling history of body snatching in Philadelphia's almshouse, and the measures taken to prevent the dissection of the city's impoverished residents. Chapter 3 examines little-known conspiracies between city officials and medical schools to appropriate the city's dead, as well as the interstate cadaver trade.

Chapter 4 demystifies body snatching, and separates myths in novels and popular culture from the reality of how body snatchers actually plied their trade. Chapter 5 covers the surprising defenses employed against body snatchers, such as grave guns, coffin torpedoes, and even cremation. Chapter 6 analyzes the relationship between body snatching and the law through William James McKnight's failed attempt at body snatching. McKnight would later become a Pennsylvania senator and be instrumental to the passage of the state's anatomy law. Chapter 7 reconstructs the history of the most infamous body-snatching scandal in Philadelphia history in 1882 that led to protests, the trial of body snatchers and Jefferson Medical College's demonstrator of anatomy, and the apparent end of body snatching in the city. The afterword considers the legacy of body snatching, and how the past informs the present controversies surrounding the treatment of human remains.

What led anatomists and medical students to go to such extreme lengths to advance medicine? Who were the "professional" body snatchers, and how did they get into the business of disinterring the dead? How did body snatching work? How did body snatchers avoid getting caught, and what happened when they did? How did the era of America's body snatchers end, and why did it go on for so much longer than in Europe? Body snatching was never just about snatching bodies: it was a window into a curious time when crime and medicine collided in America's first capital city.

CHAPTER I

"Now and Then One From the Potter's Field"

Washington Square and America's First Medical School

> The number of bodies that are allowed to go into the potter's fields throughout the country is very small, and the majority of those that reach them are not allowed to rest in them many hours. I am so positive of the truth of these assertions, that I do not consider it necessary to present any proof in support of them.
>
> —T. S. SOZINSKY, 1879[1]

In the early 1730s, a group of young, aspiring medical students met on South 2nd Street above Walnut in Philadelphia. Thomas Cadwalader was ready to share what he had learned studying medicine in England and France. At the time there were no medical schools in the 13 British colonies. Medicine was learned through apprenticeship with an experienced physician, or education abroad—for those who could afford it. None of the others, such as William Shippen, had crossed the Atlantic to learn their trade. The anticipation, not to mention the smell, must have been palpable. What they were about to do was on the cutting edge of science: an anatomy lecture.

But how did they get the body? One clue was where Cadwalader's course took place: in a building owned by none other than the chief justice of the Supreme Court of Pennsylvania. James Logan was one of Pennsylvania's most significant public officials in the early 19th century.[2] Born in Ireland, Logan sailed with William Penn on his second voyage to Pennsylvania in 1699 as his secretary, and went on to serve in a prodigious number of public offices—including mayor of Philadelphia—before he became chief justice.

A 19th-century physician observed that "so strong in those days was the feeling against dissections, to which few would have been found willing to appropriate their property."[3] Why was Logan willing to appropriate his? He was very much aware of the widespread opposition to dissection. Cadwallader Colden, who practiced medicine in the city, previously consulted Logan about a proposal for a "public physical lecture [dissection]" in Philadelphia.[4] In 1717 Logan wrote that it was "very commendable, but doubted our Assembly [the Pennsylvania General Assembly] would never go into them, that of the lecture especially."[5] As he predicted, the proposal went nowhere.

But Logan wasn't just a statesman; he was a scientist and a bibliophile who collected some of the most important scientific works of the age. He also once wrote, "Books are my disease."[6] Under English common law judges like Logan could add dissection as an additional punishment for capital crimes, such as when Hermanus Carroll was dissected by medical students in 1750 after his execution for murder in New York.[7] Like much of the early history of American anatomy, whether the body the men dissected that day was obtained legally is likely lost to history. For all we know, Cadwalader and his students were the country's first body snatchers. But what is certain is that one of Cadwalader's students that day, William Shippen, would have a son, William Shippen Jr., who would change the course of medicine as the first professor of anatomy and surgery for America's, and Philadelphia's, first medical school: the College of Philadelphia, what would become the University of Pennsylvania. Today Washington Square is a public park in Center City, Philadelphia, but in the 18th century it was a "potter's field," a graveyard for the city's marginalized groups—Shippen Jr.'s primary source of "subjects"—and where everyday people resisted the appropriation of the dead for science.

★ ★ ★

In 1758 the French and British vied for control over territory in North America in the French and Indian War. In what is now Pittsburgh, the British successfully captured Fort Duquesne from the French, where Colonel George Washington led the 1st Virginia Regiment, the last time he commanded troops under the banner of the British before the American Revolution.[8] In Philadelphia William Shippen Sr. bid a temporary farewell to his son.

The Shippens were an influential and affluent family. Shippen Sr. was a prominent Philadelphia physician, a founder and trustee of the College of Philadelphia and the first doctor hired by America's first hospital, Pennsylvania Hospital (which still operates today), and would later represent Pennsylvania in the Continental Congress. He was also in great shape and was said to have walked 6 miles shortly before his death at age 90.[9] Shippen Sr.'s grandfather Edward Shippen was Philadelphia's second mayor and had "the biggest house, the biggest person, and the biggest coach."[10]

Shippen Sr.'s son William Shippen Jr., born in the city in 1736, followed in his father's footsteps. After he graduated from the College of New Jersey (Princeton), Shippen Jr. apprenticed with his father in medicine. But Shippen Sr. wanted more for his son. He knew the value of hands-on dissection from Cadwalader's lecture, and that bodies were more readily available overseas: "But for want of that variety of operations and those frequent dissections which are common in older countries, I must send him to Europe," Shippen Sr. wrote.[11] Shippen Jr. sailed across the Atlantic in 1758, a seven-and-a-half-week voyage that was, in his words, "unpleasant and dangerous."[12] He arrived in London, the first stop in his studies, at a time of great transformation in medicine.

The modern study of human anatomy began around two centuries before, when the Brussels-born physician Andreas Vesalius published *De Humani Corporis Fabrica* (On the Fabric of the Human Body) in 1543. The book featured anatomical illustrations with unprecedented detail at a time when the understanding of the human body was based on classical texts. The work of the Greek physician Galen—backed by the Church because it conformed to religious doctrine—went unchallenged for over a millennium, but his understanding of human anatomy was hampered by the fact that he never actually performed a dissection: it was banned under Roman law. Galen instead extrapolated his findings from the dismemberment of other mammals, such as monkeys, to humans; his anatomy of the uterus was, regrettably, drawn from dogs.[13]

The Christian belief that the body needed to remain whole for resurrection limited access to the dead for dissection; body snatching and dissection was the opposite of a "proper" burial. Gradually dissection became accepted as punishment for capital offences. Vesalius was able to dissect executed criminals at the University of Padua in Italy where he taught. He also found other creative ways to obtain cadavers, like when he stole a body from a gibbet:

> A noted robber had been executed. His body had been chained to a stake and slowly roasted; and the birds had so entirely stripped the bones of every vestige of flesh, that a perfect skeleton, complete and clean, was suspended before the eyes of the anatomist, who had been striving hitherto to piece together such a thing out of the bones of many people, gathered as occasion offered.[14]

Vesalius's *Fabrica* pointed out Galen's errors and put in motion a gradual shift from the authority of classical authors to direct observation through dissection, what we would call the scientific method today.

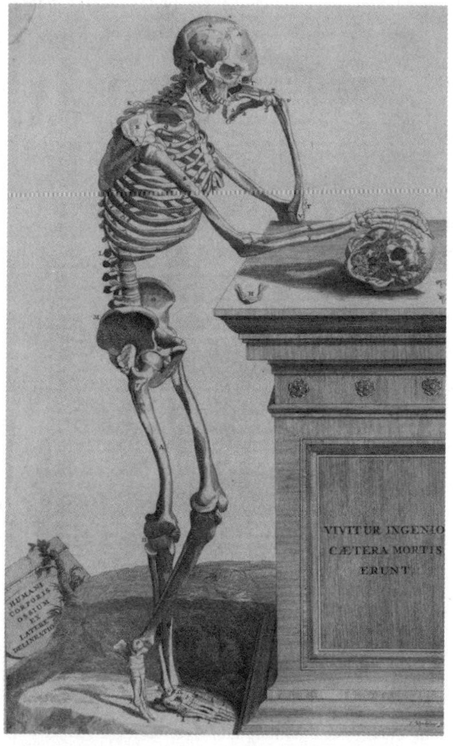

The modern study of human anatomy began with the publication of Andreas Vesalius's *De Humani Corporis Fabrica* in 1543. (Wikimedia Commons)

Until the 12th century surgery in Western Europe was performed by the clergy.[15] Monks were required by the Church to maintain a "tonsure," a haircut that left the top of the head bare, which they relied on barbers to maintain—and to assist them with surgeries.[16] But after a papal decree forbid monks from shedding blood, the barbers took their place and became barber-surgeons: they pulled teeth, performed bloodletting, and even amputations. After all, the work of grooming and surgery both required sharp tools and a steady hand.

The spinning poles you see today outside barber shops come from this history, which symbolize the practice of bloodletting, a go-to treatment for many ailments until the 19th century. The pole represents what patients held to expose their veins, and its striped, red, white, and blue colors blood, bandages, and veins (the blue color, which is unique to American barber poles, may also be a nod to the country's flag). Bloodletting was believed to restore the balance of the four "humors" that supposedly composed the human body—blood, phlegm, yellow bile, and black bile—through the removal of "impure" blood from a person's vein.

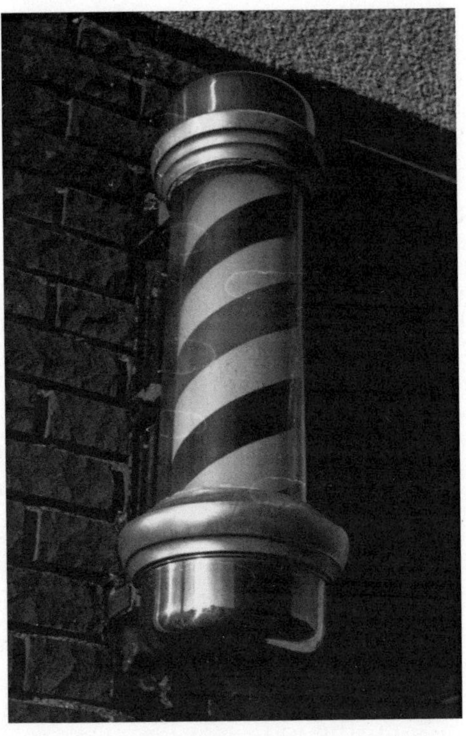

A barber pole (1984). Its colors and shape symbolize the barber-surgeon's practice of bloodletting. (Wikimedia Commons)

Medicine was an academic pursuit, and its practitioners saw themselves as above the lowly surgical trade.[17] The shift of surgery from a craft to a university-trained profession was a long, fitful process. In 1540 London's barbers joined the city's surgeons (the non-barbering kind) to form the United Company of Barber Surgeons, after which no barbers could act as surgeons, and no surgeons could act as barbers. Members were allowed to annually dissect the bodies of four executed criminals (later six), and dissection outside the company was prohibited. But when London's surgeons broke away from the barbers to form the Company of Surgeons in 1745, nothing stopped a man named William Hunter from establishing the city's first private anatomy school. Two years later his younger brother John joined him, and the Hunter brothers would become two of the century's most influential anatomists, and Shippen Jr.'s teachers.[18]

Shippen wrote about his life in London in his diary—the coffeehouses he visited and plays he attended—and in letters to his uncle: "I find the ways of Vice and Wickedness as many and as various as I expected; but can with pleasure and without boasting say, I find very little Difficulty shunning them; nothing necessary but a little Resolution and a constant call to more necessary Business."[19] But after he moved in with the Hunters in their school in Covent Garden, Shippen's days were filled with dissections: "Monday 8th. Rose at 7 dissected 7 hours, till Lecture Time at 5, after Lecture operated till 9 Supper Time under the direction of Mr. Hunter."[20]

The school made a novel offer. Following the "Paris manner" of dissection, each student would have their own body to dissect. How the Hunters obtained them was equally novel. Some came from the gallows at Tyburn, where London's criminals were executed in the 18th century. A wide range of crimes were punishable by hanging in the 18th and early 19th centuries, what became known as the "Bloody Code": over 200, including some confounding ones like "being in the company of gypsies for one month" and "strong evidence of malice in children aged 7–14 years of age." But getting bodies from the gallows wasn't easy, as family and friends of the dead fought with surgeons, sometimes violently, to prevent them from dissecting the dead.[21]

In 1752 dissection became a punishment for murder in Great Britain:

> WHEREAS the horrid crime of murder has of late been more frequently perpetrated than formerly, and particularly in and near the metropolis of this kingdom, contrary to the known humanity and natural genius of the British nation: and whereas it is thereby become necessary, that some further terror and peculiar mark of infamy be added to the punishment of death, now by law inflicted on such as shall be guilty of the said heinous offence…is hereby required…to be anatomized, or to be hung in chains.[22]

While dissection had been meted out as punishment before, the Murder Act required it, the only alternative being gibbeting (hanging in chains), in which a person was placed in a suspended iron cage shaped like a human and left out in the elements to slowly perish.[23] That gibbeting was considered an equal punishment to dissection demonstrated just how terrifying the prospect was, a fear that wasn't just for one's soul. It was a visceral fear of being physically dismembered, which probably isn't too far from how many people feel about it today.[24] The purpose of the law was to deter the crime of murder, but it also provided a more reliable supply of bodies for the Company of Surgeons (later known as the Royal College of Surgeons), like the body of Thomas Wilford, the first person supplied through the law, who grew up in a workhouse, was executed at Tyburn for the brutal murder of his wife, and dissected.[25] But the law didn't provide private anatomists like the Hunters with their own allotment of corpses, who turned to extra-legal means to meet demand.

The task fell to John Hunter, then William's assistant. John's skill in anatomy eventually outshined his brother's, but William's other achievements were considerable: he would effectively turn obstetrics (the science of childbirth) into a scientific discipline. He even served as Queen Charlotte's personal physician. Shippen would also learn "man-midwifery" in London, a task traditionally performed by women, which—like dissection—was also controversial. Now considered the "father of scientific surgery," John was also an innovator in a

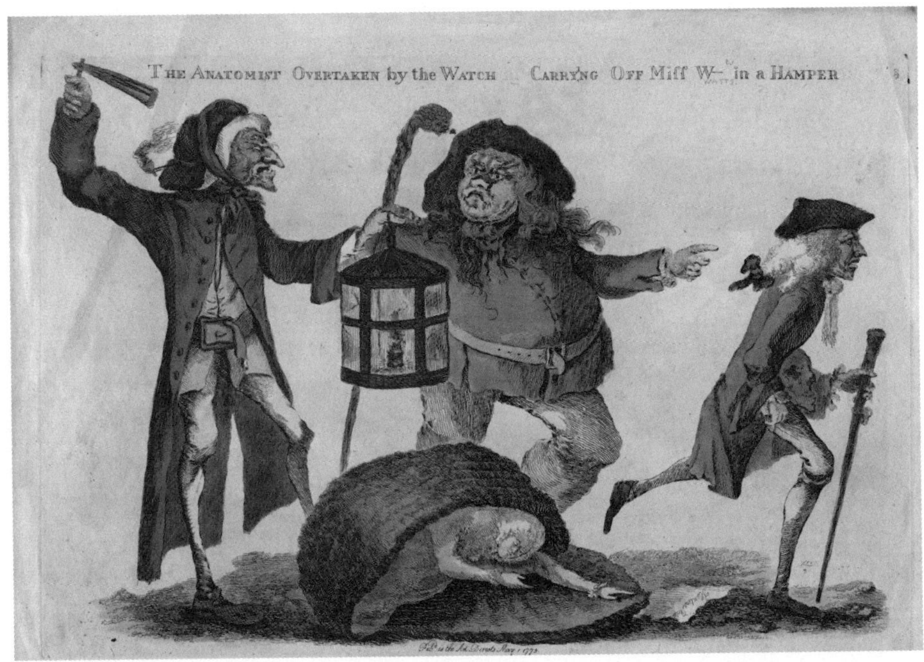

William Hunter caught red-handed in *The Anatomist Overtaken by the Watch Carrying Off Miss W— in a Hamper*, by William Austin (1773). (The New York Public Library)

complementary art: body snatching. A biographer of John noted that he probably used his own students to snatch bodies, and given the school's promise of one body per student, likely dissected with his students more bodies than any other 18th-century anatomist.[26] While London's first body snatchers were anatomists like John and his students, gangs of professional "resurrectionists" formed who fiercely competed to steal and sell the city's deceased for profit.

Joseph Naples, a member of the London Borough Gang that operated in the early 19th century, kept a diary, excerpts of which were later published. A typical night for Naples went something like this: "*Monday 27th.* At 2 o'clock in the morning got up, met the party except Dan, Went to the Big gates, got 4 Took them to Barthol, Afterwards met, took 1 to Mr. Cline, 2 to Mr. Wilson, came home. Tom & Bill got drunk, did not go out."[27] Ben Crouch became the gang's leader because of his intellect, as well as his relative sobriety compared with the others.[28] Competition got so cutthroat that warring gangs staged resurrections in their enemy's territory—leaving coffins strewn about and graves unfilled—which effectively cut off their supply because the public would demand better protection for the graveyard.[29] London's resurrectionists were so skilled that they could snatch a body in as little as 30 minutes.[30] Most victims were the city's "paupers," poor residents buried in public burial grounds.

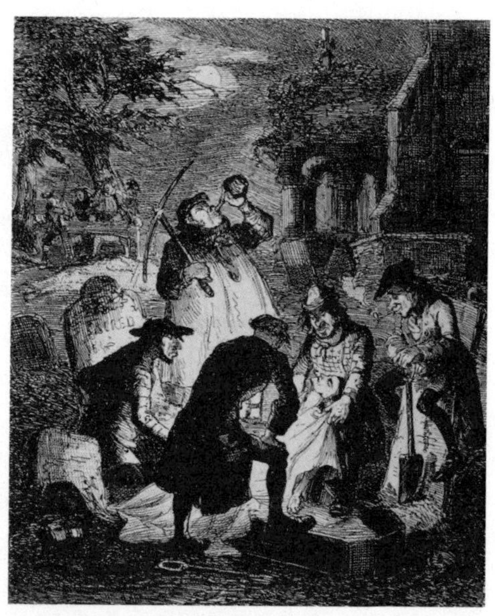

Resurrectionists, by Hablot Knight Browne (1887). London body snatchers at work. (Wikimedia Commons)

John also formed a massive collection of anatomical specimens that is on display today in London's Hunterian Museum, many of which came from victims of body snatching. One "specimen" John was determined to get was the body of Charles Byrne, the "Irish Giant" who—due to a condition known as acromegalic gigantism—grew to 7 feet 7 inches tall. Before his death at age 22 John offered to pay Charles for his body. Not wanting to become an anatomical curiosity, Charles insisted on a burial at sea so that no surgeon could get their hands on him. But after his death John paid Charles's friends for his body, which they switched out with stones in the coffin before his burial.[31] Three years later Charles's skeleton was exhibited, and until 2023 was on display in the Hunterian Museum, when it was removed from public viewing for ethical reasons. His body was not reburied at sea and is still accessible to researchers.

If Shippen didn't participate in body snatching himself as the Hunters' student, he must have at least been aware of John's nocturnal activities. After all, he lived with them. Around the time Shippen was his student, John wrote in a case book about a body they snatched from St. George's ground.[32] Before the rise of professional resurrectionists, and after, body snatching was an important skill for anatomists and their students. William encouraged his students to "speak with caution of what may be passing here, especially with respect to dead bodies," because of the sensitive nature of their studies, but likely also to keep where the bodies came from a secret.[33]

Shippen wasn't the only Philadelphian in London entangled, directly or indirectly, with the city's underground market for the dead. Founding father and renaissance man Benjamin Franklin lived in London at 36 Craven Street (near present-day Trafalgar Square), where he took daily "air baths"—sitting in his chambers with the window open "without any clothes whatever, half an hour or an hour, according to the season, either reading or writing," in his words—because he believed, not wrongly, that fresh air was good for one's health.[34] He also represented and advocated for the interests of the colonies in London, at least, until the American Revolution broke out. Shippen dined with Franklin in London during his stay; one night Franklin took Shippen to the Royal Society (the oldest scientific fellowship in the world), and another night they went to court to see the royal family and stayed up until two in the morning.[35]

In 1997, 36 Craven Street in London, Franklin's only surviving home, was being restored to turn it into a museum when a construction worker digging in the building's basement made a shocking discovery: human remains. A total of 1,200 bones from more than 15 people, including children, were unearthed.[36] Many of the bones had been cut, sawed, and a skull was even drilled. At first it was feared that the bones were evidence of a gruesome series of murders, but analysis revealed that if it was murder, it was a historical crime. The bones were dated to the mid-18th century when Franklin lived in the house, which he rented from the English widow Margaret Stevenson.

In 1770 Stevenson's daughter Mary (better known as Polly) married William Hewson, a surgeon and Franklin's friend. Now considered the "father of hematology" (the science of blood diseases), Hewson studied under and worked with William and John Hunter alongside Shippen. Hewson later entered into a partnership with the Hunters, and when it ended in a dispute, he moved into 36 Craven Street with Polly; Franklin moved into a different house owned by Margaret on the same street.[37] Franklin was scientifically inclined, most famously his experiments with electricity, but he wasn't an anatomist. The bones buried in Franklin's "basement" (what was the house's backyard at the time) were the detritus of dissections, the bodies either purchased or snatched by Hewson for the anatomy school he opened on the property after leaving the Hunters.

Hewson and his students cut the bones with scalpels, amputated them with saws, and trepanned at least one skull, and buried the evidence. Trepanning, one of the oldest known surgical procedures, has been used throughout history to reduce pressure on the brain from head injuries, or less scientifically, to let malevolent spirits out by drilling a hole in a person's head. Franklin, a curious man, was likely aware of what Hewson was up to, but probably had no direct involvement. Hewson's anatomy school, and his life, was short-lived: he died of an infection at the age of 34 after he accidentally cut himself during a dissection.

After London and the Hunters, Shippen studied in Edinburgh, another hub of body snatching, where resurrectionists like Andrew Merrilees ("Merry Andrew") inspired larger-than-life stories. In one of them, after the death of Andrew's sister, his accomplices Spoon and Mole decided to resurrect her. When the job was nearly finished—the body ready to be pulled from the grave—a ghost suddenly appeared from behind a tombstone. Spoon and Mole ran for their lives, but it was just Andrew covered in a white sheet, who then sold his own sister's body to the surgeons.[38] Most professional resurrectionists weren't known for their upstanding morals. Mortsafes, or iron cages placed over graves to prevent disinterment, from the era of the body snatchers can still be seen in Scottish cemeteries today.

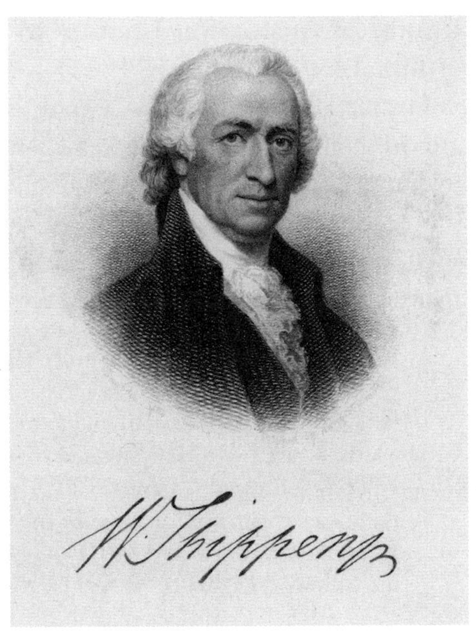

Portrait of William Shippen Jr., the first professor of anatomy for America's first medical school. (The New York Public Library)

Newly credentialed from the University of Edinburgh (where he earned an M.D.) and newlywed (while abroad he married Alice Lee, a Virginian living in London with her cousins, who perhaps admired his "handsome chiseled features"), the 26-year-old Shippen returned to Philadelphia in 1762, where he would introduce three controversial practices in his birthplace: the Hunterian approach to anatomy, body snatching, and "man-midwifery" (obstetrics). Philadelphia, and America, would never be the same.[39]

★ ★ ★

Soon after his return, Shippen met with officials from Pennsylvania Hospital bearing gifts sent by John Fothergill, a London-based physician he met during his stay, which included anatomical illustrations, a skeleton, a preserved fetus, and anatomical casts.[40] The purpose of the donation was to support medical education in the colonies. As Fothergill explained in a letter, given that "the means of procuring Subjects [bodies] with you are not easy...In the want of real subjects these [drawings and casts] will have their Use & I have recommended it to Dr. Shippen to give a

Course of Anatomical Lectures to such as may attend, he is very well qualified for the subject."[41]

Fothergill's materials were state of the art, but when Shippen publicly announced a series of lectures he had something more radical in mind: to use actual human bodies, which had never before been attempted in the colonies. There was of course Cadwalader's lecture that his father participated in before he was even born, but Shippen Jr. would be the first to do so openly, to announce it publicly in *The Pennsylvania Gazette*:

> In these Lectures the Situation, Figure and Structure of all the Parts of the HUMAN BODY will be demonstrated, their respective Uses explained, and, as far as a Course of Anatomy will permit, their Diseases, with the Indications and Method of Cure, briefly treated of; all the necessary Operations in SURGERY will be performed, a Course of BANDAGES exhibited, and the whole conclude with an Explanation of some of the curious Phaenomena [*sic*] that arise from an Examination of the GRAVID UTERUS, and a few plain general Directions in the Study and Practice of MIDWIFERY.[42]

Wielding the authority of his new credentials—which conferred the status of "gentleman"—Shippen's announcement reflected confidence, or naïveté, that he would not receive any pushback.[43] He certainly had some idea of the sensitivity of the subject, otherwise he wouldn't have also announced an introductory lecture at the Pennsylvania State House (now Independence Hall, where the Declaration of Independence and the Constitution would be signed) to explain the "Necessity and public Utility" of his lectures. While there are no surviving transcriptions of his introductory lecture, according to the notes of someone in the audience, he argued that it would advance medical progress, and invoked religion in an attempt to reframe dissection not as a blasphemous act, but one that fostered a greater appreciation of God.[44] Based on what would follow, many of his fellow Philadelphians weren't convinced.

Subsequent lectures were held in an outbuilding next to the Shippen family home on the corner of South 4th and Locust Street.[45] Shippen's course of lectures cost five pistoles, over 5,000 dollars today, and among the first 12 attendees was a young Benjamin Rush, later a signatory of the Declaration of Independence (now considered the "father of psychology").[46] Rush found Shippen's lectures engaging and informative.[47]

They also weren't strictly for education, but the "Entertainment of any Gentlemen, who may have the Curiosity to understand the ANATOMY of the HUMAN FRAME," as the advertisement for it read.[48]

The earliest known body the students dissected was an enslaved Black man found "with a Piece of a Glass Bottle under him, with which he had cut his Throat in such a terrible Manner... after the Coroner Inquest had pronounced him guilty of Self Murder, his Body was immediately ordered, by Authority, to Dr. Shippen Anatomical Theatre."[49] He wouldn't be the last. There were similar newspaper reports of enslaved Black men who took their own lives sent to Shippen in the years that followed. At the time suicide was legally equivalent to murder, and while Shippen and his students used the body for science, they were effectively punishing resistance to slavery, and setting an example for others.

Macabre stories swirled around Shippen's house, which still stands today, and its outbuilding, at the time and long after. In one of the city's earliest histories, John Fanning Watson wrote that Philadelphians expected the school to "fill the peaceful town with disquieted ghosts."[50] It was "always shut up" and "had 'No Admittance' for ever grimly forbidding, at the door," and students came and went "in the shades of night."[51] As for the bodies, after dissection the "flesh was boiled, and their bones burnt down for the use of the faculty!"[52] Less plausibly, Watson wrote that "from the great chimney about once a fortnight issued great volumes of black smoke, filling the atmosphere all the country round with a most noisome odour—offensive and deadly as yawning graves themselves!"[53] More likely was Watson's claim that a graveyard was later discovered on the property. After all, the body parts had to be buried somewhere.

Some let their imaginations run wild: "It was further suspected that he kept vats in which he disposed of the bones and fragments of the bodies, and there was a superstition which associated these imaginary receptacles with such deeds as Macbeth's witches performed when they gathered around the cauldron."[54] Poems even circulated about the school:

> And awful stories chain'd the wondering ear
> Or fancy led, at midnight's fearful hour,
> With startling step, we saw the dreaded corse [corpse]![55]

The body-snatchers! they have come
And made a snatch at me;
It's very hard them kind of men
Won't let a body be!
Don't go to weep upon my grave
And think that there I be
They haven't left an atom there
Of my anatomy![56]

The last poem Watson attributed to Shippen's house was actually a shorter version of one written by English poet Thomas Hood called "Mary's Ghost. A Pathetic Ballad":

'Twas in the middle of the night,
To sleep young William tried,
When Mary's ghost came stealing in,
And stood at his bed-side.

O William dear! O William dear!
My rest eternal ceases;
Alas! my everlasting peace
Is broken into pieces.

I thought the last of all my cares
Would end with my last minute;
But tho' I went to my long home,
I didn't stay long in it.

The body-snatchers they have come,
And made a snatch at me;
It's very hard them kind of men
Won't let a body be!

You thought that I was buried deep,
Quite decent like and chary,
But from her grave in Mary-bone
They've come and boned your Mary.

The arm that used to take your arm
Is took to Dr. Vyse;
And both my legs are gone to walk
The hospital at Guy's.

I vow'd that you should have my hand,
But fate gives us denial;
You'll find it there, at Doctor Bell's,
In spirits and a phial.

As for my feet, the little feet
You used to call so pretty,
There's one, I know, in Bedford Row,
The t'other's in the city.

I can't tell where my head is gone,
But Doctor Carpue can:
As for my trunk, it's all pack'd up
To go by Pickford's van.

I wish'd you'd go to Mr. P.
And save me such a ride:
I don't half like the outside place,
They've took for my inside.

The cock it crows—I must be gone!
My William, we must part!
But I'll be yours in death, altho'
Sir Astley has my heart.

Don't go to weep upon my grave,
And think that there I be;
They haven't left an atom there
Of my anatomie.[57]

Philadelphians were suspicious of Shippen and made their displeasure known, most often by throwing stones and breaking windows, but that was tame compared with what would follow three years later.[58]

In 1765 John Morgan, a Philadelphian who graduated from the University of Edinburgh just a year after Shippen, petitioned the College of Philadelphia to establish the first medical school in the colonies. Shippen discussed the idea with Morgan when they crossed paths in London, and likely also with Fothergill, who described Morgan as Shippen's "able Assistant" in the endeavor.[59] But Morgan made the petition without consulting Shippen, and received all the credit for establishing the first medical school in British North America, and becoming its first professor of medicine.

Adding salt to the wound, in a speech at the college's commencement that year Morgan dismissed surgery as a "mechanical art," unlike the study of physic (medicine), that could be taught merely through apprenticeship; he also denied that Shippen had the idea of opening a medical school at all.[60] Even in the second half of the 18th century many still viewed surgery as beneath the profession, as if they were still no better than barber-surgeons. But surgeons would have the last laugh: today it is one of the medical field's most prestigious and highest-paying specializations. Despite Morgan's contempt, Shippen became the college's first professor of anatomy and surgery, and set the record straight in his letter of application, when he claimed that he was just waiting for Morgan to return from Europe before he proposed the creation of a medical school.[61] But Shippen would never forget Morgan's slights, and it was the start of a feud that would escalate to the point that it impacted the ability of the Continental Army to function during the Revolution.

In 1765 *The Pennsylvania Gazette* announced the opening of the first American medical school in Philadelphia. To cultivate "Medical Knowledge in America," the Medical Department of the College of Philadelphia offered lectures on anatomy and physic.[62] At the time a license wasn't even required to practice medicine in colonial America.[63] "Quacks" abounded: in 1775 residents of Northampton County, Pennsylvania, complained about doctors whose care caused unnecessary deaths.[64] Before the professionalization of medicine, which the College of Philadelphia pioneered, anyone could claim to be a physician. Aspiring doctors would also no longer have to travel to Europe to learn medicine. Instead, many would travel from around the country to study in Philadelphia. From the opening of the college to the late 19th century, physicians with degrees gradually assumed functions previously performed by midwives and traditional healers, and the study of anatomy in particular set the medical profession apart from others and cemented their authority over medical and surgical matters.[65]

Shippen's announcement started innocently enough, but then it took a dark turn:

> It has given Dr. Shippen much Pain to hear, that notwithstanding all the Caution and Care he has taken, to preserve the utmost Decency in opening and dissecting dead Bodies, which he had persevered in, chiefly from the Motive of being useful to Mankind, some evil minded Persons, whither wantonly or maliciously, have reported to his Disadvantage, that he has taken up some Persons who were buried in the Church Burying Ground, which has distressed the Minds of some of his worthy Fellow Citizens.[66]

Given how few bodies were legally available for dissection, it wasn't surprising that Philadelphians questioned Shippen's sources. Philadelphia only executed nine people in the 1760s.[67] Shippen was the first to face a dilemma that would bedevil all anatomy instructors that followed: too many students and not enough bodies. Shippen's response to his fellow Philadelphians wasn't exactly reassuring. While it's possible he took bodies from a white churchyard, he had to know that would draw too much attention. Shippen's defense wasn't that he didn't take bodies from cemeteries, but that he took the *right* kinds of bodies:

> The Doctor, with much Pleasure, improves this Opportunity to declare, that the Report is absolutely false; and to assure them, that the Bodies he dissected, were either of Persons who had willfully murdered themselves, or were publickly executed, except now and then one from the Potters Field, whose Death was owing to some particular Disease; and that he never had one Body from the Church, or any other private Burial Place.[68]

Churchyards were off-limits, but Shippen believed he was allowed to dissect condemned bodies—murderers and suicides—a right based on precedent rather than law. This right didn't extend to taking other marginalized bodies buried in the potter's field, but he wouldn't have publicly acknowledged doing so if he didn't think he could get away with it. Dissection as punishment for capital crimes would later be explicitly established in American law. The "Potters Field" referred to Washington Square, known then as Southeast Square, a public burial ground near Independence Hall. The "potter" in potter's field is a reference to grounds that were suitable for local potters to dig clay, but little else, and is also referenced in the Bible.

Today Washington Square is a public park, one of the four public squares William Penn envisioned for his "greene country towne" nestled between the Schuylkill and Delaware rivers, but it didn't start out that way.[69] The city's initial plan included no cemeteries.[70] The deceased were buried by denomination, usually next to places of worship. But as Philadelphia's Common Council stated, a burial ground was needed "for all strangers or others who might not so convenient [*sic*] be laid in any of the particular enclosures appropriated by certain religious societies to that purpose," which the square became in 1706.[71] In other words, it was a public graveyard for individuals unable to afford a "proper" burial and "strangers," unidentified people, and other outcasts from society.

Later, enslaved and free Black people, barred from white churchyards, interred their dead there. The square was racially segregated; Black and white people were buried separately. Washington Square was more than just the primary burial place for 18th-century Black Philadelphians. According to a 19th-century history of Philadelphia, it was also a place of cultural activity, referred to as "Congo Square":

> It was the custom for the slave blacks, at the time of fairs and other great holidays, to go there to the number of one thousand, of both sexes, and hold their dances, dancing after the manner of their several nations in Africa, and speaking and singing in their native dialects, thus cheerily amusing themselves over the sleeping dust below!...going to the graves of their friends early in the morning, and there leaving them victuals and rum![72]

But once medical schools started opening, the square could also be a source of fear:

> Among the negroes it was a superstition in almost every household. It is said that they would walk far out of their way at night time in order to avoid Washington Square when it was [a] Potter's Field or that if they had to pass it they would run as fast as their heels would carry them. Some of them even believed that the doctors or their students laid plans for decoying people into their rooms, quietly slaying them and then pickling the bodies for future use! Many a doctor noted how, when a negro met him walking along the streets at night, the negro would look at him askance or dart out of the way, as if he feared that he might be made a victim of the doctor's mysterious cunning.[73]

But Black Philadelphians made Washington Square their own, and vigorously defended it from body snatchers. Some buried in Washington Square likely died of "some particular Disease" as Shippen suggested, especially during epidemics, but what he really meant was that people buried in the square weren't entitled to a dignified interment, to rest in peace.

In the 17th century burial with a headstone wasn't common, except for the wealthiest, but as graves became more individualized in the following century, an anonymous, unceremonious interment in the potter's field became stigmatized.[74] Washington Square was a resting place of last resort, isolated on the then-edge of the city, a place where most Philadelphians would have dreaded being buried.[75] The land was not ideal for burial; it was uneven, and a stream flowed through part of it.[76] An even greater mark of dishonor than burial in the potter's field was body snatching and dissection.

Care for the dead took many forms, religious and secular, in particular times, places, and cultures, but had three components: the preparation of the body for burial, the transportation of the body to the grave, and finally, its interment.[77] In 18th-century Philadelphia death was a familial affair that took place in the home among family, friends, or neighbors.[78] The same was true of medical care for the sick and injured, but only wealthy Philadelphians could afford the services of physicians.[79] Burial in churchyards was the norm, and never too far from the living, as most could not afford carriages and would walk to funerals.[80] For Protestants and Catholics generally, women "layed-out" the dead, by washing, positioning, and dressing the body to make them presentable.[81]

All faiths accepted the importance of caring for the dead. For Jewish Philadelphians, the body was an object of reverence, yet also unclean; rather than family performing the ritual preparation of the body, it was performed by local specialists or charitable groups, and burial was expected to occur rapidly.[82] Mikveh Israel, the first Jewish cemetery in Philadelphia, was established in 1740; Jews had been present in the Philadelphia area prior even to the city's founding.[83] While there is little recorded history of African burial practices in Philadelphia, 17th-century Africans on the Gold Coast (West Africa) also washed and clothed bodies, and placed objects within and on top of graves.[84]

While in biological terms life and death are mutually exclusive, after death but before burial the body was sometimes seen as being in an intermediate state between life and death in which the "human corpse possessed both sentience and some sort of spiritual power."[85] Disturbing the dead in this state was seen as imperiling one's soul, and there was no higher humiliation of the dead than the desecration of the corpse—even for medical purposes—because it violated fundamental beliefs and practices of care for the dead.[86] The dead have a power and specialness, one that transcends even religion.

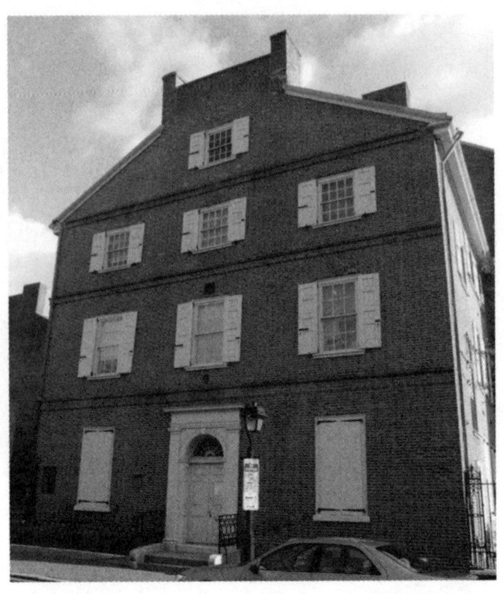

The Shippen family home in 2013, the site of the first anatomy lecture and anatomy riot in the colonies. (Wikimedia Commons)

Curiously, the Shippen family home was built just blocks away from Washington Square around 1750. The land was disagreeable, but it was a perfect location for easy access to a graveyard and to avoid prying eyes. But if Shippen thought he could get away with taking bodies without opposition, he was in for a rude awakening. One day in 1765 Shippen was in the middle of a dissection when he heard a crash outside. An unruly crowd of people had gathered who, believing he was in the carriage parked in front of the property, broke its windows with stones. Someone even fired a musket ball where Shippen would have sat. The unfortunate coachman driving the carriage fled from the "shower of missiles," and fearing for his life, Shippen fled as fast as he could through an alley.[87] It was the first of many "anatomy riots" that would follow in America.

The incident known as the "sailor's mob" may have been sparked when Shippen disinterred a sailor named Jack in Washington Square for dissection. A 1789 poem by Francis Hopkinson recounted the event:

> Methinks I hear them cry, in varied tones,
> "Give us our father's—brother's—sister's bones."
> Methinks I see a mob of sailors rise—

> Revenge!—revenge! they cry—and damn their eyes—
> Revenge for comrade Jack, whose flesh, they say,
> You minc'd to morsels and then threw away.[88]

Philadelphia's port was central to the city's economy, and most were employed by it in some way; sailors had an especially high mortality rate but low pay, so they were usually buried in the potter's field, a fate they would have rather avoided.[89] A story that circulated in 1785 demonstrates this well: the bones of a man were found by sailors on a ship at port in Philadelphia, which were then interred in the potter's field.[90] But the ghost of the man, agitated over his burial in such a lowly place, haunted the ship's sailors and identified the sailor who killed him; the accused denied the charges, but many believed the supposed ghost over the man.[91] Burial in the potter's field was upsetting, apparently even to ghosts, but body snatching and dissection could drive people to violence.

Many medical schools experienced riots similar to Philadelphia's, and some were far more lethal than the sailor's mob, such as the 1788 "Doctors' Riot" in New York City. Exactly how the riot was sparked was uncertain, but in one telling a young surgeon jokingly waved a dismembered arm he was dissecting at a group of young boys playing outside New York Hospital. The student told one of the boys that the arm was his mother's, who recently passed away. The boy, shaken, rushed to tell his father, who had his wife's body exhumed to see if there was any truth to the student's "joke." Sure enough, her grave was empty. The father, his "fellow-workmen," and a crowd that formed around them stormed the hospital, where they wreaked havoc on the institution's collection of bones and specimens.[92] Medical students were spared violence only because the police arrested them for their own protection.

Unsatisfied, the next day a crowd made their way to the steps of Columbia College, the city's only medical school, where founding father Alexander Hamilton failed to persuade the mob from entering. They found nothing incriminating in the college, or in the houses of local physicians they searched after. Finally, the mob of thousands, massed at the jail where the students were being held, chanted "Bring out your doctors! bring out your doctors!" and attempted to break in: "They then smashed in the windows with stones…but the handful of men inside

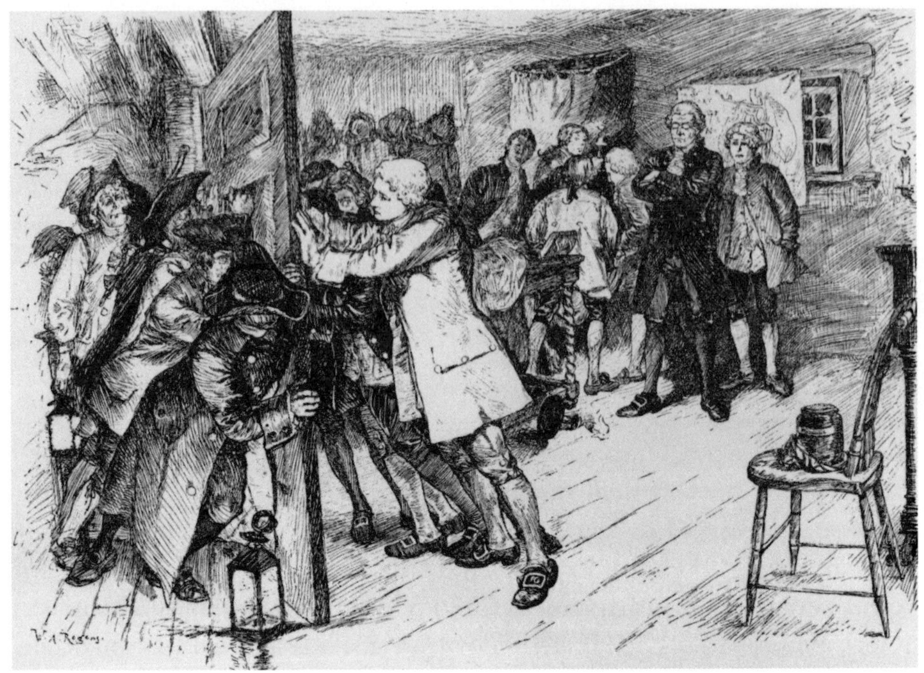

An Interrupted Dissection (1882), a depiction of New York City's 1788 Doctors' Riot. (Library of Congress)

took possession of these, and, with such weapons as they could find, beat them back."[93] The militia was called in, and when the crowd threw bricks and stones at them—founding father John Jay among them—the soldiers fired on and attacked the crowd with bayonets.[94] Multiple militiamen and rioters lost their lives, and more were injured.

In 1770, five years after the sailor's mob, Shippen responded to similar allegations of body snatching in *The Pennsylvania Gazette*:

> Many of the inhabitants of this City, I hear, have been much terrified by sundry wicked and malicious Reports of my taking up bodies from the several Burying grounds in this Place…I [declare that I] never have had, and that I never will have, directly or indirectly, one Subject from the Burying ground belonging to any Denomination of Christians whatever. Having been informed that two Families were very lately much terrified, by unkind Insinuations, that their deceased Friends would not rest in their Graves…it was generally believed I had taken up a young Lady from Christ Church Burying ground, whose Grave has been opened within these few Days, and her Body found in its sacred Repository undisturbed.[95]

Reading between the lines, it's clear Shippen believed burying grounds not "belonging to any Denomination of Christians" were fair game. While Christians were certainly buried in Washington Square, Shippen's message was that if someone wasn't buried in a churchyard—even if they would have been if they had the choice—they didn't have a legitimate claim to be left in the grave. In addition to an unnamed young woman, he denied dissecting Elizabeth Roberts, but felt it necessary to get a signed document from the physician who treated her before her death to prove it. At the suggestion that his students were body snatchers, Shippen included an affidavit—made before the mayor of Philadelphia—from one of his students:

> And secondly, that scarce any one doubted but I had in my Theatre the Body of Elizabeth Roberts, who formerly lived as Housekeeper with William Lyons, Esq; this Woman, as Dr. Kearsley jun. (who attended her in her last Illness) has given me from under his Hand, died in the Middle of Summer of a putrid Fever, yet no one doubts but I dissected her in the Middle of Winter...none of your House, or Kindred, shall ever be disturbed in their silent Graves, by me, or any under my Care. As it has been insinuated, that Subjects might have been brought from these Burial Places by my Pupils, without my Knowledge, I have added an Affidavit of Joseph Harrison, Student of Medicine, who has lived in my Father [*sic*] House ever since I began my anatomical Lectures, and who has had an Opportunity of knowing where every Body was obtained, that ever I dissected in America.[96]

We'll probably never know for sure if these accusations were true, but it showed that most Philadelphians didn't trust Shippen: the young woman's grave was opened to confirm that she still rested in peace. In 1769 Christ Church, where Benjamin Franklin's grave can be visited today, built a wall made of stone around its cemetery.[97] In 1770 two executed criminals from Gloucester, New Jersey were sent to Shippen by "order of the Chief Justice," perhaps because all the attention from the controversy made obtaining bodies secretly more difficult.[98]

When the American Revolution broke out in 1775 the suspicion around Shippen stopped. In times of war, body snatching was unnecessary: corpses were plentiful. The battlefield was its own kind of medical school, and despite the tragic human cost of war, many important medical breakthroughs have emerged from conflict. George Washington's

Revolutionary War mandate for Continental Army soldiers who had not already been infected to be inoculated against smallpox may have altered the course of the war by staving off the spread of the deadly disease, an early demonstration of the effectiveness of immunization campaigns. In 1777 John Adams wrote to his wife Abigail about his visit to Washington Square, where thousands of American soldiers ravaged by smallpox and other diseases were buried:

> I have spent an Hour, this Morning, in the Congregation of the dead. I took a Walk into the Potters Field, a burying Ground between the new stone Prison, and the Hospital, and I never in my whole Life was affected with so much Melancholly. The Graves of the soldiers, who have been buryed, in this Ground, from the Hospital and bettering House, during the Course of the last Summer, Fall, and Winter, dead of the small Pox, and Camp Diseases, are enough to make the Heart of stone to melt away.
>
> The Sexton told me, that upwards of two Thousand soldiers had been buried there, and by the Appearance, of the Graves, and Trenches, it is most probable to me, he speaks within Bounds. To what Causes this Plague is to be attributed I dont know...Disease has destroyed Ten Men for Us, where the Sword of the Enemy has killed one.[99]

Later that year the British occupied Philadelphia, the capital, where the Continental Congress convened. During that time soldiers from both sides were buried in the square, including American soldiers who were subjected to terrible conditions in Walnut Street Jail; the occupation ended the following year, an effort that provided little military advantage for the British.[100]

Like medical education, medical care still had a long way to go in the 18th century. Depending on the nature of the injury, some soldiers' wounds, from musket shots to bayonet wounds, were "treated" with amputation: before anesthetics or antiseptics, soldiers had to endure the pain of losing a limb and the high likelihood of dying of infection after. Even in the Civil War amputation would be the most common procedure surgeons would perform. When it came time for General George Washington to choose a second director general to oversee the Continental Army's hospitals (what today we would call the surgeon general of the United States Army), his first choice was the eminent Shippen, but Congress chose Shippen's nemesis: John Morgan.[101] The first director general, Benjamin Church Jr., was fired after he turned out to be a spy for the British.

But when Shippen was put in charge of a hospital in New Jersey the following year, Morgan believed Shippen was angling for his position, and Washington wrote that the conflict that ensued between them had worsened medical care for soldiers in 1776.[102] Shippen and Morgan's personal vendetta couldn't have helped the war effort, especially when the lives of soldiers and the outcome of the war were at stake. Morgan was fired from his job; Shippen took his place and faced the same problems as Morgan, such as supply shortages, bad organization, personal conflict, and an unhelpful Congress.[103]

It was Shippen whom Washington ordered to inoculate all soldiers that passed through Philadelphia: "Necessity not only authorizes but seems to require the measure, for should the disorder infect the Army in the natural way and rage with its usual virulence we should have more to dread from it than from the Sword of the Enemy."[104] At the instigation of Morgan and Benjamin Rush (Shippen's former student who became Morgan's supporter), Shippen faced a court martial for a wide range of charges, including negligence and fraud, but was acquitted on all counts. He resigned from his position.

★ ★ ★

On September 17, 1787, the Constitution of the United States was signed in present-day Independence Hall in Philadelphia. About three months later, a block away from the birthplace of America, a very different scene unfolded in Washington Square. As William Shippen Jr. wrote in a letter to his son:

> We have been & are still at a great loss for want of a subject for dissection & demonstration, few die & the negroes have determined to watch all who are buried in the Potters [*sic*] field—the young men have been twice driven off by arms, once fired on & 2 wounded with small shot, on Saturday night with the assistance of 6 invalids with muskets they beat off the negroes & obtained a corps [*sic*] & I lodged it in the [anatomy] Theatre.[105]

After the war Shippen returned to teaching, but he faced strong resistance from Black Philadelphians in the new republic who sought to protect, gain control of, and legitimate their longstanding burial place of Washington Square. Black Philadelphians took the defense of their dead into their own hands and instituted a cemetery watch, and were armed and ready to defend Washington Square from the "young men," Shippen's students. One 1906 newspaper claimed that Shippen taught his students not just the art of anatomy, but body snatching.[106] Shippen's students were fought off twice and wounded in the process, and only secured a body with the assistance of six "invalids" in the fight, veterans injured during the Revolutionary War who joined in the third shootout.

Just two years later a poem by Francis Hopkinson, writing with Philadelphia in mind, seemed to allude to the same or a similar event:

> THINK how, like brethren, we have shar'd the toil
> When in the Potter's Field we fought for spoil,
> Did midnight ghosts and death and horror brave
> To delve for science in the dreary grave—
> Shall I remind you of that awful night
> When our compacted band maintain'd the fight
> Against an armed host? fierce was the fray
> And yet we bore our sheeted prize away.[107]

But Shippen didn't get away with it that night. He took the body to his home, but then, "The resolute impertinent blacks broke open ye house stole ye subject & reburied it— This transaction was made known to ye friends of the dead who joined ye negroes in great numbers on Sunday night & swore death and destruction to ye Faculty."[108] Black Philadelphians broke into Shippen's home to take back the body. Many Philadelphians—"friends of the dead"—did not take Shippen's side and condemned the College of Philadelphia's faculty. It wouldn't be the last time.

In another letter soon after, Shippen wrote to his son:

> After 10 days peace I procured a subject from the Bettering house [almshouse] as secretly & properly as it was possible but no sooner had Beatly & Clark put it in at the back window of the Theatre...they were met by 15 or 20 blacks armed (who patrol every night around the Potters [*sic*] field & down our street & I saw them) no other way could they be discovered...the blacks broke 2 locks entered ye Theatre brought out the body paraded it before the door, crossed the alley and buried it in the Potters [*sic*] field. I say they determined I shall not

> have a subject this winter. We have no police in this city to correct this lawless proceeding, & 9/10th of the citizens join or countenance these black devils—'tis difficult to find out in ye night who they are, and if I would prosecute them to punishment my house and life might answer for it.[109]

Even if he successfully took a body, there was the chance that it could be taken back by force. Shippen's inability to respond to multiple break-ins in his own home demonstrated just how precarious his situation was. The Board of Wardens managed the night watch, which alerted constables of nefarious doings by ringing a bell they carried, but it's unclear whether they patrolled Shippen's home on the edge of the city.[110] But based on his own estimation, most Philadelphians—even the night watch—probably supported leaving even those buried in the potter's field in their graves. Yet Shippen seemed to believe that the law was on his side, that theirs was a "lawless proceeding," and that he could "prosecute them to punishment." In reality, he operated in a gray area of law and popular opinion and had little recourse.

Black Philadelphians used force to protect Washington Square, but also democratic processes. It had been seven years since Pennsylvania's General Assembly passed "An Act for the Gradual Abolition of Slavery" in 1780, the first abolition act adopted by any democracy in the world. "Gradual" was the key word: it freed no one initially, only children born after the law was passed, when they reached the age of 28. With limited options for employment, land, or even security, freedom wasn't much different from slavery in Philadelphia, and full abolition only came in 1847.[111] Enslaved Africans were taken by force to Philadelphia even before the city's founding, by the Dutch, Swedes, and the English; William Penn owned 12 enslaved Africans, and William Shippen Sr. two in 1774.[112]

In 1782 free Black people petitioned for the erection of a fence around their section of Southeast Square, presumably to ward off body snatchers.[113] In 1787 the Free African Society was formed, the first nondenominational benefit mutual aid society for Black Philadelphians; one of its functions was to pay for members' burials.[114] In 1790 the Free African Society petitioned to rent Southeast Square and, in 1791, to erect a church in Washington Square, which was one of the first political actions undertaken by the Black Philadelphia community.[115] The number of free Black people who lived in Philadelphia would continue to grow and become a burgeoning community by the following century.

Shippen may have gone to such extreme lengths to obtain bodies because of his zeal for medical progress, but that wasn't the only reason. One was economic: Shippen made money directly from student fees, although it wasn't his only source of income.[116] Without cadavers, he couldn't teach, which risked his status as a fount of anatomical knowledge. He was able to get away with it by the implicit assent of elite Philadelphians to appropriate bodies from the potter's field. Careful to not cross racial or class lines and take so-called "respectable" bodies, Shippen—one of the most influential Philadelphians—leveraged his social standing as a gentleman to dissect the city's marginalized groups.[117] But he didn't always avoid the suspicion of elite Philadelphians.

While Washington Square was targeted most frequently, no cemetery in the city was truly safe, even respectable ones. When a body was taken from St. Peter's in 1779, they later raised funds to build a brick wall.[118] A 1788 Philadelphia newspaper noted:

> The Theatre for dissecting dead bodies has become such a terror to the citizens... friends of deceased persons are now watching the Friends [Quaker] burial-ground. On Monday night three persons crossed from the College yard into the burial-ground, who were followed...and got off. Tuesday night the watchman, in his round, was asked by an unknown person, if the burial-ground was watched... Should there unjustifiable acts be committed, and the citizens fortunate as to detect any person or persons in the fact [*sic*], that they be held up to public resentment.[119]

Shippen would doubtless have received more widespread opposition if he took bodies indiscriminately. Even today Philadelphia ghost tours that include Washington Square mention the ghost of Leah, a Quaker woman who protected the potter's field from body snatchers, supposedly spotted by a Philadelphia police officer in 1994.[120]

In the 1790s Shippen's anatomical lectures were moved to a location only a block away from Southeast Square: Surgeon's Hall near South 5th Street above Walnut.[121] In 1791 the College of Philadelphia merged with the University of the State of Pennsylvania to become the University of Pennsylvania. When the College of Philadelphia moved to its 9th Street campus, Shippen's dissections continued in Surgeon's Hall to not draw unwanted attention to a still-controversial practice, which was, like his home, in a remote location.[122] But finally, in 1807, the 9th Street building was expanded to include an anatomical theater where Shippen gave his last introductory lecture; he died the following year at the age of 71.[123]

In 1793 over 1,300 victims of yellow fever, a virus transmitted by mosquitoes, were buried in Washington Square, after which the potter's field was said to be at full capacity; in all the epidemic killed 5,000 people, 10 percent of Philadelphia's population. Many of the city's wealthy residents and its leaders fled, including George Washington, who blamed his wife: "It was my wish to have stayed there longer; but as Mrs Washington was unwilling to leave me amidst the malignant fever which prevailed, I could not think of hazarding her & the Children any longer by my remaining in the city."[124] But physicians like Benjamin Rush stayed behind, although his treatments, such as bloodletting, likely harmed more than they helped. The following year Washington Square ceased to be a burial ground and transformed into its originally intended purpose: a public park, which it remains today. While it is possible that some of the bodies buried there were relocated, many still reside there today. In 1805 the University of Pennsylvania sought to expand onto Washington Square.[125] If it had gone through, the university would have for a time been housed above the graves of the burial place its own anatomist had plundered.

In Washington Square today, signs describe the history of the square as a potter's field, and the many Philadelphians and others who were interred there. The Tomb of the Unknown Revolutionary War Soldier, the most visible landmark in the park, memorializes the soldiers buried there in mass graves. No sign mentions Washington Square's role in the history of medical education, or body snatching. Shippen's house, now referred to as the Shippen-Wistar house (Caspar Wistar succeeded Shippen as professor of anatomy and surgery), is now privately owned and not open to the public. A historical marker outside the building mentions only Wistar, not Shippen, and nothing about body snatching.

As Philadelphia became the center of American medicine in the following century, the medical community needed a larger source of bodies to sustain its rapid growth. Just as burial in the potter's field was stigmatized,

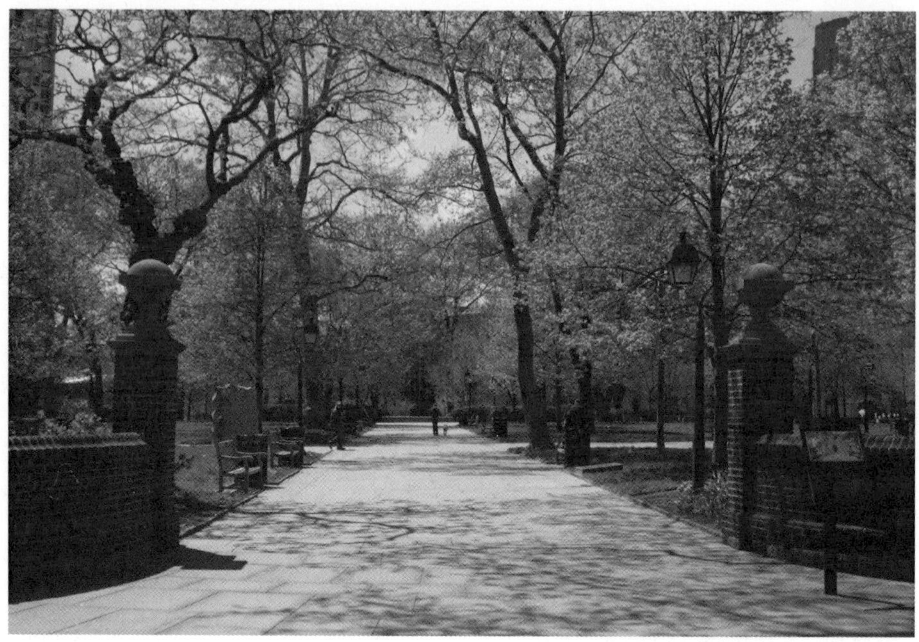

Washington Square in 2013. Formerly a potter's field, it's now a public park. (Wikimedia Commons / CC BY-SA 4.0)

so was dying in public institutions like Philadelphia's almshouse, which was where anatomists looked next. Justified by classist ideas and the delegitimization of the poor's right to a "proper" burial, body snatching and dissection of almshouse "inmates" became institutionalized. At one point, the almshouse's board became known as the "Board of Buzzards" that preyed on the dead bodies of the poor. The almshouse was also a significant source of anatomical specimens displayed in museums like the University of Pennsylvania's Penn Museum and Mütter Museum, which have been the subject of recent controversies. Body snatching would grow to a scale that few, including Shippen, could have imagined.

CHAPTER 2

"Board of Buzzards"

Dissecting the Destitute at Blockley Almshouse

> Poverty, misfortune and sickness, universally regarded as evils, yet counterbalanced by yielding, as fields for scientific observation, a rich harvest of solid, practical medical knowledge.
>
> —DAVID HAYES AGNEW, 1862[1]

In 2001 construction workers building a parking garage in West Philadelphia discovered something unexpected: human remains. Archaeologists tasked with excavating the site near the University of Pennsylvania could only estimate the number of bodies they eventually unearthed. A total of 442 people were found in individual graves with coffins stacked eight deep or in pits, and parts of at least 248 people were buried in boxes mixed with syringes, plates, and bottles.[2] The macabre trove was a mystery until its source was located on a historic map: Blockley Almshouse's burial ground.[3] That wasn't all that was uncovered; so was the sordid history of how poor relief became entangled with the expansion of medical education, and body snatching, in 19th-century Philadelphia.

Almshouses were public institutions that provided impoverished people with food, shelter, clothing, and even healthcare, but at a terrible cost: freedom.[4] Blockley's inhabitants, referred to as "inmates," received life's basic necessities in exchange for grueling work. Conditions in Philadelphia's underfunded and overcrowded almshouse were appalling. The starving Oliver Twist famously said, "Please, sir…I want some more," to the workhouse master in Charles Dickens's novel of the same name, but in London—and Philadelphia—the reality was far worse. From May 1775 to May 1776, "147 Men, 178 Women, and 85 Children, were admitted as Poor, most of them naked, helpless and emaciated with Poverty and

Disease to such a Degree, that some have died in a few Days after their Admission," to Philadelphia's almshouse.[5]

In the 18th century Philadelphia pioneered American medicine, but in the 19th it became the center of the field. The American Medical Association was founded in the city in 1847, the largest professional society of physicians and medical students in the country today. Philadelphia was the leading publisher of American medical journals and textbooks.[6] The city produced many of America's first doctors, with enrollment exceeded only by Paris and Edinburgh.[7] Philadelphia's almshouse was a dreaded last resort for its residents, but not for resident physicians who treated the sick in the institution's hospital.

Blockley was an early example of a teaching hospital where medical students and recently graduated resident physicians gained practical experience treating the sick. But what was best for medical education was not necessarily what was best for relief of the poor. In life inmates were subjects of clinical instruction attended by the city's medical students. In death they were subjects of anatomical instruction and used to prepare specimens for anatomical museums, collections that still exist today.

Philadelphia was a destination for medical students, in no small part because of bodies available for dissection, as featured in an 1833 Jefferson Medical College advertisement: "[Philadelphia's] hospital and alms-house are large institutions...they afford to the pupils who attend the lectures delivered in that city, the best opportunities for clinical study. The supply of subjects for dissection is abundant even to profusion."[8] In 18th-century Philadelphia, body snatching was small-scale and sporadic, centered on Washington Square, but as the number of medical schools grew exponentially around the country in the following century—from four in 1800 to over 160 by 1900—so did body snatching, centered on Blockley.[9] The history of the Philadelphia Almshouse is the story of how the poor became institutionalized, and fueled the rise of America's "City of Medicine," and body snatching, in the 19th century.[10]

★ ★ ★

Before William Penn embarked on the ship *Welcome* in 1682 for his first voyage to Pennsylvania, he wrote in a letter, "Pity the distressed and hold out a hand of help to them; it may be your case; and as you mete to others God will mete to you again."[11] Penn's words became a reality in his new colony in 1705 when the Pennsylvania Poor Law, modeled after the English Poor Laws, established a system for poor relief to assist Philadelphia's poverty-stricken populations.[12] Caring for the poor was a local responsibility: counties established Overseers of the Poor to collect taxes to pay for "outdoor" relief, such as food, clothing, and money.[13] But the aid came with conditions. To prevent all but the neediest from seeking assistance, starting in 1717 recipients were required to wear the letter "P" for "pauper" on their shoulder. Failure to do so was punishable by having "relief suspended or withdrawn, and also to be whipped and kept at hard labor for twenty-one days."[14]

Groups like Penn's Religious Society of Friends, better known as Quakers, also cared for their own. The Friends' Almshouse was established in 1713, which was actually a few houses that could fit one or two destitute, widowed, elderly, or sick members:

> They were one story in height, with a garret room and a great tall chimney... The situation was secluded and peaceful. Trees and shrubbery ornamented the grounds, and the inmates devoted themselves to the cultivation of flowers and medicinal plants. It was a place of calm seclusion, partitioned off from the noise and bustle of a city, and it afforded to the inmates opportunities for study and meditation, while at the same time they could follow such light occupations as were suited to their age and weakness.[15]

In the early 1730s Philadelphia opened its own almshouse to administer "indoor" relief. As the Philadelphia Common Council explained, "The Poor of this City Dayly Increasing, it is ye opinion of this Council that a Workhouse be Immediately Hired to Imploy poor p'sons, and Sufficient p'sons appointed to keep them at Work, And the House & psons be Provided by the Overseers of the Poor."[16] The city's almshouse was a single home built of brick and open to all Philadelphians, located between 3rd and 4th, and Spruce and Pine Streets in what is now Center City, Philadelphia.

Such responses to poverty, whether private or public, reflected colonial America's social system of family and kinship: outdoor relief supported the poor in their homes, while indoor relief housed them in a home-like environment.[17] But even in these early years the institution was plagued by corruption that would lead to far graver abuses of power: there were complaints "against Overseers of the Poor who have supplied the poor with necessities out of their own stores and shops at exorbitant prices, and also against Overseers who have paid unreasonable accounts to their friends and dependents for services done the poor."[18]

By 1767 the city's almshouse was overcrowded and unable to accommodate the rising numbers of the "lower sort." A new solution was proposed by Quaker merchants: using private funds to pay for a new, expanded almshouse.[19] In exchange for their donations, the affluent merchants—incorporated as the "Contributors to the Relief and Employment of the Poor in the City of Philadelphia"—elected members of the Board of Managers that ran the public institution.[20] That same year the almshouse moved to a complex that was then the largest building in British North America, with two L-shaped wings, one for the almshouse and one for the workhouse that were attached to a central building, between 10th and 11th, and Spruce and Pine Streets.[21] Philadelphia's first two almshouses were built on the then-edge of the city, not far from Independence Hall; their very existence decreased surrounding property values.[22]

The shift in care from a home-like setting to an institution, and from outdoor relief to indoor relief, also reflected a shift in attitudes toward the poor. Poverty was viewed not as a problem of circumstance, but character: there were the moral, "industrious" poor, down on their luck, and the immoral, "idle" poor, supposedly more likely to commit crime.[23] Benjamin Rush wrote that the morals of the poor were more important to society than their well-being.[24] While officially known as the Philadelphia Almshouse and House of Employment, its nickname—the "Bettering House"—embodied the broader mission of the merchants who funded it: moral reform.

Able-bodied residents were put to work repairing and making shoes, weaving, and carpentry, among other tasks, controlled and disciplined with uniforms and daily regimens, in an effort to "better" their character.[25] The forced, unpaid labor was supposed to turn the "undeserving" poor into self-sufficient members of society, and to turn a profit to help fund the institution. Benjamin Franklin echoed the widespread sentiment at the time when he wrote, "the best way of doing good to the poor, is not making them easy *in* poverty, but leading or driving them *out* of it."[26] But the causes of poverty were economic, not moral, such as rapid population growth, immigration, and the aftereffects of the Seven Years' War.[27] Instead of facilitating rehabilitation, the almshouse only fostered resentment.

Children admitted to the almshouse were also indentured to receive an education or learn new skills, and not just orphans. David Jacobs, a nine-year-old boy, was separated from his mother and "bound out" for 12 years to a man to learn a trade, but was instead forced to work as a chimney sweep until almshouse authorities discovered the scheme and cancelled his indenture.[28] Those unable to work resided in the almshouse, or if they were sick, the hospital, like the 24-year-old Rhodah Coombes. Admitted to the almshouse in 1800, she was married to a shoemaker named William Coombes, who abruptly left her. Without money or friends and suffering from a serious illness, unable to work, she was admitted to the almshouse.[29]

The most populous group of almshouse residents were native-born white people, but their numbers—along with native-born Black people—gradually decreased as immigration increased.[30] Black residents were placed in the worst wards and areas of the almshouse and likely experienced higher death rates as a result, but all residents experienced the institution's terrible conditions. A 1784 report revealed that "shocking abuses prevailed" in the Bettering House, where "It was ascertained that all kinds of unwholesome food, including 'maggotty butter,' had been served to the inmates."[31]

The almshouse's first burial ground was Washington Square; over 120 inmates were buried there in 1790.[32] To reduce expenses, inmates were later tasked with building coffins and burying their fellow residents. In 1787 an employee of Walnut Street Prison, adjacent to Washington Square, found a way to profit from his position: by charging the almshouse to bury its dead.[33] John Reynolds refused to open Washington Square's gate until he received, as he put it, "fence money." The Board of Wardens, which managed the square, ended the extortion, but Reynolds was able to keep his ill-gotten gains. That same year William Shippen Jr. wrote in a letter to his son that he "procured a subject from the Bettering house as secretly and properly as it was possible," the first known body snatching in the almshouse.[34]

After Washington Square became a public park, the Bettering House buried its dead in a graveyard farther southwest where, around 1822, Philadelphians living near it complained about its condition. Pits were dug that could fit up to four coffins stacked on top of each other. Until the pit was full it was only lightly buried, but that could take over a month, "*in consequence of the many visitors*...[who] *carry off the corpses left there for interment*...which certainly makes it very offensive to have all the corpses for that length of time nearly exposed to the open air."[35] An almshouse committee investigated and discovered an empty coffin in one of the pits and recommended that the bodies be buried individually: "persons who are desirous of having corpses ought to have some trouble to obtain them, instead of having them placed above ground and inviting persons to carry them away to save the trouble of burying them."[36] The responsible party was censured, but graveyard attendants continued to make "*arrangements with the doctors as they please*."[37] It wouldn't be the last time almshouse authorities attempted to stop body snatching and failed: the institution would become notorious for it.

By 1788 many of the wealthy merchants who funded the Bettering House went bankrupt during the Revolution, and the Overseers—renamed the Guardians of the Poor—took over management of the institution. Again, due to overcrowding the almshouse moved to its final, larger location on a farm across the Schuylkill River, between 34th Street and University Avenue, in 1835. "Old Blockley," as it would later be known (for the township it resided in), included an orphanage and even an insane asylum, in addition to an almshouse, workhouse, and hospital, segregated by sex and race. Blockley was uncharitably described at the time as a "seething mass of infirmity, disease, vice and insanity."[38] Blockley's architect was William Strickland, one of the two architects for Philadelphia's Eastern State Penitentiary that still stands today, where Al Capone once resided.

Inmates suffering from psychosis faced especially bad conditions: "They were placed in dark, close and damp cells in the eastern wing, and the medical gentlemen did not seem to trouble themselves very much about them. They appeared to think that insanity was incurable, and even the mildest cases were in cages like wild beasts," and even put in chains.[39] In an area set aside for women with mental health issues, 17 were killed by falling walls in 1864, caused by structural issues that were introduced with the addition of heating in the building.[40] In 1885 the Insane Department burned down, which killed 19 inmates;

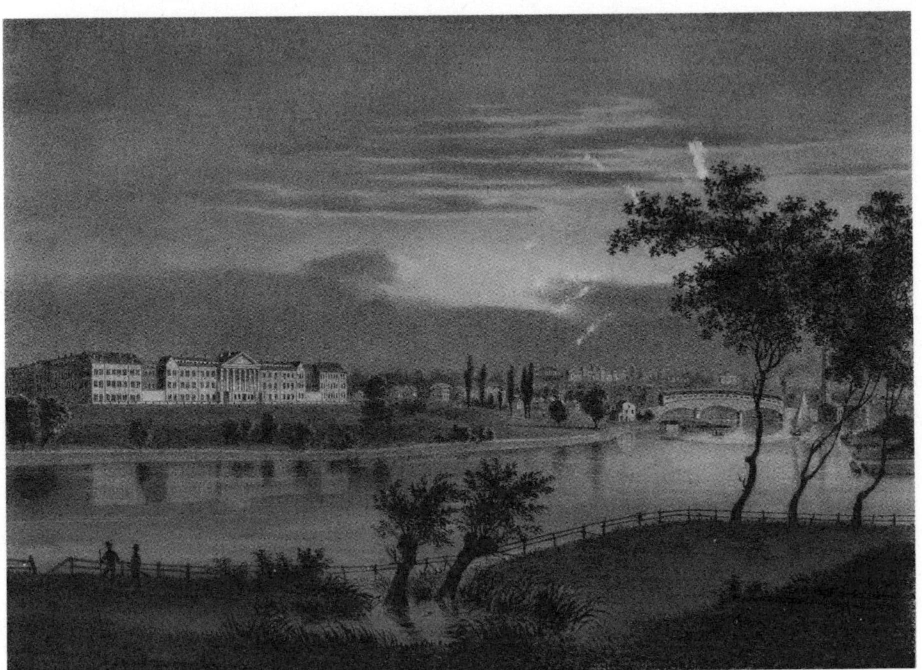

Old Blockley, Philadelphia's third and final almshouse, located in West Philadelphia above the Schuylkill River. (Library of Congress)

the department lacked even basic fire safety infrastructure for the time, such as fire escapes or even a fire extinguisher.[41]

While it was hoped that the workhouse and farm would generate profit to make the poorhouse self-sustaining, corruption, bad management, and overcrowding left the institution chronically underfunded.[42] Over time, the public's view of the poor grew more critical; as a result, Blockley's function shifted away from the Bettering House. It began to focus not on rehabilitation, but pure institutionalization—or, to paraphrase historian Roger D. Simon, being put in prison simply for being poor.[43]

Blockley's complex was built with high walls and fences surrounding its buildings and grounds to prevent residents from escaping.[44] Blockley's isolation in what was then a rural area of West Philadelphia was of course no accident, and served to separate inmates from Philadelphia proper. Instead of being seen as "deserving" or "undeserving," almshouse residents were more frequently blamed for their condition, which shaped their treatment—in life and death.[45]

History of the Philadelphia Almshouse

Name	Established	Location	Cemetery
Philadelphia Almshouse	Early 1730s	Between 3rd and 4th, Spruce and Pine Streets (Center City, Philadelphia)	Washington Square
Philadelphia Almshouse and House of Employment ("Bettering House")	1767	Between 10th and 11th, Spruce and Pine Streets (Center City, Philadelphia)	#1 Washington Square #2 Between 11th and 12th Streets, Christian Street and Washington Avenue[46]
Blockley Almshouse ("Old Blockley") Philadelphia Hospital	1835	Between 34th Street and University Avenue (West Philadelphia)	#1 Between Locust and Spruce, 32nd and 33rd Streets #2 South side of 34th Street, east of S. University Avenue[47]
Philadelphia General Hospital	1902–77	Between 34th Street and University Avenue (unchanged) (West Philadelphia)	South side of 34th Street, east of S. University Avenue

Since it first opened, the almshouse had a hospital, officially named Philadelphia Hospital after the move to Blockley. Its earliest known physician was William Shippen Sr., and Shippen Jr. later practiced there as well and wielded considerable influence, to the point that his recommendation was enough to secure someone a position.[48] Some of the most important physicians of the time practiced in Blockley, such as Thomas Bond, Benjamin Rush, Philip S. Physick, William E. Horner, Joseph Pancoast, David Hayes Agnew, and Samuel D. Gross. The almshouse's hospital opened earlier, but Pennsylvania Hospital (located near Independence Hall) is generally considered America's first hospital because, unlike the almshouse which performed many functions, it was dedicated solely to medical care.

Both Philadelphia Hospital and Pennsylvania Hospital became important teaching hospitals, where medical students and newly graduated resident physicians put into practice what they learned in the classroom, which is standard today. However, Philadelphia Hospital was more central to medical education because it was the city's largest and busiest hospital.[49] Pennsylvania Hospital's admissions criteria were also more restrictive: it only admitted those judged to be among the "deserving" poor with a treatable condition; patients even had to leave a deposit for burial in case of death.[50]

18th- and 19th-century hospitals were deathtraps before it was understood that germs caused disease: basic hygienic practices like washing hands, bed sheets, or surgical instruments that decreased the likelihood of infection were not followed. As one Blockley resident physician told it, the operating room and table were made of wood, a highly absorbent material where germs flourished, but at that the time "surgical cleanliness or antisepsis was unknown."[51] If surgical instruments were dropped, they were not sterilized, and surgeons wore their uniform on average for a year without washing it, which was about as clean as you would expect—not at all: "Nothing healed by first intention unless the intention of the operator was thwarted by a kind providence, and good luck won in spite of our efforts."[52] The almshouse's hospital facilities always left much to be desired—Blockley's first operating room didn't provide enough light or ventilation, and the clinic room was originally not directly connected to the hospital, so inmates had to be moved in all kinds of weather between buildings.[53]

Mortality after surgery was so high that Blockley's surgeons sometimes refrained from operating "even though the patient may be suffering under a mortal disease, sure to destroy life if no operation is performed."[54] At the time it was more common to administer care in the home, which was probably for the best, but Philadelphia's poor had limited options: "no sick man or woman sought its walls willingly. It was the last resort for those who could not gain admission to other hospitals, or who were absolutely friendless and penniless," as a Blockley resident physician explained.[55] Like burial in the potter's field, living or dying in the almshouse was a mark of shame. As one almshouse superintendent was known to say, "Once a pauper, always a pauper."[56] The stigmatization and vulnerability of almshouse inmates created unique opportunities, and conflicts of interest, for Philadelphia's medical community.

While in 1766 Thomas Bond inaugurated the first clinical lectures in America in Pennsylvania Hospital, in 1770 students of "good character" were allowed to attend America's first obstetrical clinic in the Philadelphia Hospital and observe cases of labor.[57] Resident physicians were permitted to practice in the Bettering House starting in 1788, "on trial, and a committee was appointed to frame suitable regulations for their government," after heated debate among the almshouse's managers.[58] A former almshouse superintendent noted, "When this was inaugurated many persons considered it as a rather dangerous innovation, as medical students were surrounded by an atmosphere of mystery and suspicion at that period."[59] In 1803 clinical instruction for medical students began in the almshouse, on the condition that instructors were responsible for keeping students in line.[60]

The almshouse's administration was right to be concerned about misbehaving medical students and resident physicians. University of Pennsylvania medical students were accused of misbehavior, using dead bodies without permission, and other violations of Pennsylvania Hospital's norms.[61] In 1834 a resident physician was forced to resign for "a violation of the rules of the house in relation to the examination of the dead" in the almshouse.[62] Once a resident physician threw the contents of a tumbler in an almshouse superintendent's face, and later threw the entire tumbler at him, a fight that ended with the young physician being restrained while trying to grab a fire poker. After this incident the resident physicians were warned that "their continuance in the institution depended upon their conducting themselves in a more decorous manner."[63]

The almshouse's managers were also uneasy about the dissections that physicians performed. According to a Blockley surgeon:

> Students at this time were regarded with no small amount of suspicion; and even at the present time there are not wanting many persons who entertain toward them a good deal of reserve and distrust. It is a shocking thing, gentlemen, to cut up dead people; and one might suppose from the horror with which some people shun you, that students were in the habit of eating them.[64]

Another term for body snatchers was "ghoul," an evil spirt that not only stole the dead, but also feasted on them. Dissection was a rite of passage, a shared experience that inducted students into an anatomical fraternity, a culture marked by macabre humor, sometimes involving the dead bodies they dissected, and alcohol-fueled merriment.[65] Membership came with certain obligations. Dissection required secrecy: students could face expulsion for disclosing information, such as the source of bodies, and instructors and other staff were expected to be similarly circumspect.[66] It was a transgressive culture that didn't exactly endear physicians to their almshouse colleagues, or the wider community for that matter.

At first dissection also generated unease among medical students. After Joseph Leidy's first dissection in the 1840s as a student at the University of Pennsylvania, he didn't return for six weeks.[67] Such a reaction was not unusual. Another Philadelphia medical student in 1853 described how he overcame his initial unease. Dissection hardened his heart to the point of callousness, a kind of clinical detachment.[68] Leidy would later become Penn's professor of anatomy.

Resident physicians treated almshouse inmates in life and used them for instruction, as Blockley resident physician Arthur Ames Bliss vividly recalled in his memoir. He recounted the moments leading up to an operation on a certain Anderson the "Bum" in 1883:

> [He was] wheeled into the operating room this morning. In the great amphitheater, the circling rows of seats were crowded with students, tier above tier, until, to one standing down in the deep arena, the very air above seemed filled with eager faces. The patient lay on a high, revolving, wooden table in the centre of the

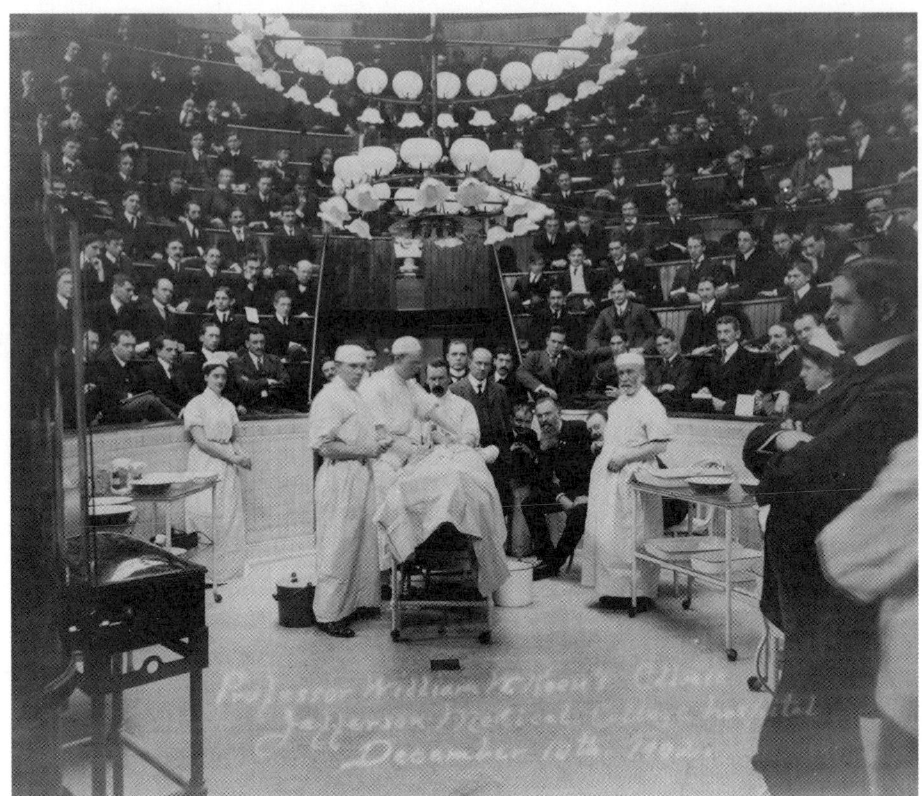

Professor William W. Keen's Clinic, Jefferson Medical College Hospital, December 10, 1902. Similar to what Anderson the "Bum" would have seen in Blockley's operating room. (Library of Congress)

> arena, and was clearly displayed in the light which streamed from the skylight in the lofty roof. Close by stood Dr. P., knife in hand, lecturing to the students in his rather stagely manner.[69]

It's not difficult to see how this could make inmates uncomfortable or even be detrimental to their health. The use of almshouse inmates for instruction was controversial, and the feelings of inmates themselves were a concern of almshouse authorities not always shared by physicians. An 1845 Blockley Hospital Committee reported that "None of the patients are exempt from the liability of being thus exposed [in the lecture room]," and that "There are rights possessed even by the recipients of charity which should be guarded, and feelings which should be respected."[70]

There was widespread fear among inmates that they would be used as "clinical material" in lectures.[71] Surgeries were performed in front of other patients until a dedicated space was provided for that purpose in the early 19th century.[72]

In an era before informed consent, inmates had little say over the course of their medical treatment and had to trust that physicians made decisions that were in their best interest. But administering the best patient care was not the exclusive focus of resident physicians, who were also trying to further their budding careers and were often more interested in unusual or unique medical and surgical cases.[73] Almshouse residents were subjects of medical experimentation, according to almshouse surgeon David Hayes Agnew: "if a patent medicine was to be tested, or any charlatan maneuver to be practised, the Philadelphia Hospital was the field in which the trial was to be made."[74] By virtue of being in the almshouse, inmates were at the mercy of physicians, a power disparity that was sometimes exploited, in life and death.

Bliss also described how he felt about Edmunds, an inmate he dissected:

> But there was no need of this care for Edmunds' clay [body]; his friends long ago lost to him; his family, criminals themselves, indifferent as to his fate; not even a dumb animal to care for him or mourn his loss! All that remained was soon accomplished, and he has found rest at last, after his twenty-five years of tossing and stumbling and suffering through his vagrant and criminal life, in the ash heap of the Potter's Field.[75]

Bliss seemed to be trying to justify Edmunds's dissection to himself, as if he didn't believe that the body of this "crime-possessed pauper," as Bliss put it, was just "clay" to be freely used for science.[76] But if other physicians shared Bliss's doubts, that didn't stop them from using almshouse residents as they saw fit. Clinical detachment, a transgressive anatomical fraternity, and perceptions of almshouse residents as immoral, idle, and criminal led to the rise of body snatching in Blockley, which by 1845 was rampant. It was the same year the Guardians of the Poor who managed the almshouse protested "the practice of taking the bodies from the graveyard to the Lecture rooms" that had plagued the almshouse for years.[77]

★ ★ ★

There was always tension between the Guardians and physicians because of their conflicting visions for the almshouse. For the Guardians, the purpose of the almshouse was relief of the poor. Regardless of how flawed their understanding of almshouse residents was and how to best help them, the Guardians looked after their best interest as they saw it. In addition to treating the sick, physicians viewed the almshouse as a site to train the next generation of doctors and for medical research, but what was in the best interest of advancing medical science was not necessarily in the best interest of inmates' health.

By 1828 instruction in the almshouse or Pennsylvania Hospital was a requirement for graduation from the University of Pennsylvania, and students purchased admission tickets directly from lecturers, until they became free around 1860.[78] Practicing in a teaching hospital had become so essential to medical education that students couldn't graduate without it. The importance of the almshouse to the medical community became clear whenever it was threatened. When the almshouse moved to West Philadelphia in 1835, the University of Pennsylvania was still located in Center City, and physicians worried the move would imperil Philadelphia's national standing in medical education by making its most important teaching hospital less accessible. Physicians also complained that there were "many important pecuniary [financial] interests of the citizens which would be materially injured by a measure curtailing the means of medical instruction."[79]

The Guardians' response was that medical instruction was secondary to treating the sick, and one physician called their reasoning "a splendid masterpiece of colossal stupidity, and proves that among the governors of the institution there must have been then, as there usually have been since, individuals who had attained the last possible degree in the way of being asses."[80] But when the almshouse moved, medical students followed, transported to Blockley by horse-drawn omnibuses and by ferry. In 1872 Penn's campus relocated to West Philadelphia next to the almshouse on land purchased from Blockley, and in 1874 established its own teaching hospital, the Hospital of the University of Pennsylvania, the first hospital run by a university in the United States.

As medical education rapidly expanded in the 19th century, in Philadelphia and America at large, more students required more bodies, and physicians looked for ways to justify the dissection of almshouse residents, to deny them the dignity in death that other Philadelphians enjoyed. Anatomy was central to medical education at the time, as direct knowledge of the human body through dissection granted physicians authority over the treatment of the human body. The ability of students to dissect would have been expected, and supply issues would have disrupted this aspect of students' education. A common argument of the time, and one made by Blockley physicians, was that "as paupers are of no use to society while living, there is no wrong done in making them useful when dead."[81] It was a justification rooted in the same ideas that led to the institutionalization of the poor in the first place. The destitute could pay back their debt to society—as if they were criminals—if their bodies could be used to advance medical progress.

The Guardians rejected the idea that all residents of almshouses were of "no use" to society while alive or responsible for their situation, that some were once industrious members of society who had fallen on hard times or become sick.[82] While still distinguishing between types of impoverished residents, the Guardians pushed back against blaming the poor as a whole for their plight, and expressed a belief that all deserved the same care after death afforded to others:

> Few, and perhaps none, are so deadened in feelings as not to desire the rites of Christian burial, for who would not revolt at the idea, if they were consulted on the subject, of permitting their bodies to be exposed in the lecture rooms, cut to pieces for the benefit of the schools and then thrown into a pit containing the remains of hundreds of others.[83]

Despite this, the Guardians allowed the dissection of one type of inmate: the "unclaimed." Before burial, deceased inmates were kept in the "dead house," which was strictly regulated:

> An official is constantly stationed to guard it, and rules of the most stringent character have been adopted for the safe keeping of the bodies and to preserve them unmutilated in cases where the friends of the deceased can be found. A messenger is always dispatched forthwith to inform the relatives or friends of the deceased, in order that they may have an opportunity of removing the body.[84]

As the Guardians explained, "We are not the foe of science. For this reason we cannot oppose the relinquishment to the medical colleges of the bodies of those who die at the public charge, without friends whose feelings might be lacerated by the circumstances."[85] In other words, if there were no family or friends who claimed an inmate for burial, then no one would be emotionally distressed by their dissection, and there would be no harm, no foul. But the innocuous-sounding designation of "unclaimed" disguised its true purpose: the wholesale appropriation of the bodies of the poor for medical education.

In order to claim an inmate, family or friends had to pay for their burial, but given that only the most desperate were admitted into the almshouse, their loved ones likely couldn't afford it.[86] The almshouse could have just made it so that anyone who died without relatives or friends were available for dissection, but requiring relatives to claim them all but assured that the poor would be dissected by default, regardless of the feelings of relatives or inmates themselves.[87] Inmates knew that body snatching was widespread in the almshouse and worried about what would become of their remains after death. None would have willingly allowed their body to be dissected, a fate normally reserved as punishment for murderers. According to the Guardians:

> Burial here, during the lecture season, is a mockery, and to be buried elsewhere is some times asked as the last and greatest favor...And may not this anxiety to have the remains cared for and protected after death be partly produced by the idea that the spirit may continue to be cognizant of what is done to the mortal part? *That death does not mean a total disconnection?*[88]

Physicians accused the Guardians of "mawkish sentimentality," that the bodies of the poor were "mere matter"—or "clay" as Bliss put it—that there was no connection between the body and the soul after death. Opposition to dissection represented the triumph of "superstition" over anatomists' "enlightened" views, but most Guardians, or the wider public, did not agree with them.[89] The "unclaimed" designation was a much more subtle, and effective, way to dissect most of the residents who perished in the almshouse.

Blockley's first burial ground was located in the space now occupied by Franklin Field, a sports stadium on the University of Pennsylvania's campus that was used until around 1860.[90] While the claimed would presumably be buried anywhere other than the almshouse's graveyard, the institution continued to bury some of its unclaimed dead, but they didn't stay there for long, if they even made it to the graveyard. The management of the dead-house didn't instill much confidence. A history of Blockley described how "The man who had charge of the dead-house had illuminating episodes of alcoholic exaltation, which were among the most remarkable that I had ever witnessed, and presented strong suggestions of the alcohol from broken specimen bottles."[91] According to a Blockley resident physician:

> It would seem that there must be some natural connection between dead-house men and spirits, for I remember that one winter...the river was full of ice, and the dead-house official of the time not clearly distinguishing between it and terra firma, plunged into the water and was drowned. His body was brought to the house the next day.[92]

Another manager of the dead-house was "Cadaverous Charlie," as a resident physician called him, a "cheerful-tempered" German man, who didn't appear to be an alcoholic but had a curious way of sizing up the people he met:

> He never estimates a man, either living or dead, by his face or reputation, but judges of his worth by considering what kind of a skeleton he would make, if the fortunate opportunity offered. A stranger at once excites his notice, and he exclaims, "Mein Gott! Vhat a vine skeleton dat man vould make!" Or, it may be that the whole *ensemble* was below standard, and that the skeleton would be a frank failure and unsatisfactory.[93]

Physicians obtained bodies from the dead-house, the graveyard, or any part of the almshouse they could. There were too many cases of body snatching in the almshouse to claim that the Guardians played no role, if only passive, in its persistence. The Guardians accepted the flawed logic that if physicians only dissected unclaimed bodies, no harm would be caused, which ignored the feelings of family and friends who couldn't afford to claim inmates, and the feelings of inmates who were powerless to stop it. The Guardians also agreed that the snatching of almshouse inmates from the potter's field was preferable to snatching from "respectable" graves: the threat of body snatching by physicians in the wider community warranted allowing the same physicians to dissect the almshouse's inmates instead. Ultimately, physicians succeeded in normalizing body snatching in the almshouse. The Guardians disagreed with physicians on points, but not their ultimate effect: the exploitation of the almshouse's deceased. For an institution always seeking to cut costs, it made sense: why pay for burial with public funds when bodies could be dissected for free? Some would even be sold for profit.

When the conflict between physicians and the Guardians came to a head it wasn't over body snatching. Inexperienced resident physicians were said to be running the hospital with little supervision.[94] A Blockley resident physician described his position as one of authority, a power that often went to their head: "Our relations with all under-officials, nurses, and pauper inmates were almost those of masters and slaves. After living in such circumstances for several months we became naturally overbearing, dogmatic, and, it must be confessed, more or less brutal. We met the slightest curtailment of our rights with indignant protest."[95]

The almshouse's medical department was dogged by mismanagement and negligence, accusations that the Guardians also faced. After a female almshouse employee complained about the "deportment and language" of resident physicians during mealtime in 1845, they were reprimanded for "violations of propriety."[96] In response, the physicians refused to administer medical care, and were dismissed and replaced for this dereliction of duty.[97] A different kind of violation of propriety soon followed, when "two members of the Board happening to enter an unfrequented, and, as they supposed, an unoccupied part of the building, discovered the mutilated remains of a human body, in a condition too revolting to be described. Appearances indicated that the remains had been there for several months, and we suppose they had been overlooked."[98]

There was further trouble later that year when a cockroach scurried across the table where the resident physicians and steward took their meals, which was squashed without "due formality and decorum" (by whom was unclear).[99] The physicians demanded to take their meals at a different table, which was denied, and they resigned in protest, which disrupted medical care for inmates. As a result, instruction for medical students was not allowed in the almshouse for nine years by the Guardians. Medical instruction was halted in the almshouse for almost a decade not by body snatching, but a cockroach. Instruction returned to the almshouse in 1854, but in 1856 clinical instruction stopped again for two years due to conflict between the Guardians and the chief resident physician.[100] Finally, students returned in 1858, and so did body snatching.

In 1856 Dr. Mosely, a member of the Guardians, was accused of selling the bodies of dead almshouse residents. An almshouse investigation revealed that 21 bodies were unaccounted for after comparing almshouse death and burial records. The almshouse committee that investigated blamed this disparity on shoddy record-keeping, not body snatching. Pieces of paper were placed on coffins with the name of the deceased, which often fell off and were lost, the only record of the burial conveniently missing. The chairman of the committee was censured by the Guardians and prevented from making a "minority report," possibly because it would have revealed that a Dr. Mosely was selling bodies, and only recommended that better records of burials be maintained. The accusation against Dr. Mosely was never proven, and newspapers vilified the Guardians for "stifling" the inquiry. After this the Guardians became known as the "Board of Buzzards," perceived as vultures who preyed on almshouse bodies—defined by either their inability to stop body snatching or their outright complicity—who "stole the roof off of the Almshouse."[101]

Blockley's second graveyard was near what is now the University of Pennsylvania:

> [It is] surrounded on three sides by a close board fence, and on one, the east, by a pale-fence, in the centre of which is a gateway. The fences, and the cemetery in general, have a somewhat dilapidated appearance...In all the enclosure, but one grave is marked—a solitary wooden tablet, with a brief inscription. Built against the board fence on the north side is a home-made hut about twelve feet long and half as many feet in width, the abode during the daytime of a one-legged Argus, who guards these sacred precincts.[102]

In 1860 Philadelphians living around the graveyard were concerned about body snatching. The "ferryman" (who previously operated the ferry across the Schuylkill River) who managed it was "a man of very low character" and "charged from ten to fifteen dollars [to medical students in the winter] for each human subject for the dissecting tables, and a brisk business is done during the terms of the college lectures in the corpses of those who die at the Almshouse and whose bodies are not claimed by friends"—money that he pocketed.[103] The administration was unable to fire the ferryman due to his connections. Mr. Linnard, a member of the almshouse administration, was more upset that the ferryman profited off the sale of bodies, that the money didn't go to the almshouse, not the sale of the bodies themselves.

In response to uproar over more cases of body snatching, in the early 1860s the Guardians finally took action to stop the body snatching of *all* inmates, including the unclaimed, in the cemetery. One of the Guardians expressed the desire to have all almshouse bodies given the "same care and protection as is given to those who have friends and relatives to watch over and guard their last resting places."[104] The almshouse's graveyard was completely unprotected. One Guardian suggested requiring a permit to enter the graveyard.

But the Guardians resolved to do something far more radical: build a receiving vault to "deposit and keep the remains of those who die in the Almshouse, until removed by their friends or their graves rendered secure from violation by reason of the partial decomposition of their bodies."[105] In other words, if bodies were claimed they would be buried by family or friends, not on the premises, and all others—probably the vast majority—would be buried only after decomposition had rendered their bodies useless for dissection. Such were the extreme measures necessary to safeguard the almshouse's dead. The structure was completed in 1862, with a capacity of 42 coffins, and a watchman was already stationed nearby. The almshouse put the management of the vault into the hands of an almshouse superintendent.

This development worried the medical community. In an article published in a medical journal at the time, a physician attempted to rewrite not only history, but the present. The "prejudice" against dissection had given way to "more rational and enlightened views," and the vault was just an overreaction to "popular clamor" by the Guardians over "some improprieties, or indelicacies, or indiscretions."[106] The body snatchers, physicians who circumvented misguided popular attitudes toward dissection, were a thing of the past, but if they couldn't dissect the almshouse's "unclaimed" then physicians would be *forced* to steal bodies.

Certainly, they argued, there was nothing wrong with dissecting the almshouse's unclaimed, who had no friends or family who would be upset by it. But that was just a convenient cover for dissecting nearly all of the almshouse's bodies.

The almshouse's vault threatened to end the Philadelphia medical community's primary supply of bodies, but the Guardians backtracked. The pressure from the medical profession must have been greater than that from the public, because they decided to not use the vault during the "warm weather," which effectively allowed body snatching to flourish unchecked.[107] An 1879 issue of *Penn Monthly* noted:

> In 1862 the Guardians of the Poor of the city and county of Philadelphia, in their wisdom did resolve that they would no longer allow bodies to be carried away for dissection; but, through the influence of more sensible men, they were prevailed on not to put the resolution in force.[108]

Instead of ending body snatching, the vault was a stark reminder that any defense of the dead would be circumvented.

According to a member of the Board, after the vault had been rendered useless in 1862:

> The speaker had been informed by the watchman on the bridge [crossing the Schuylkill River towards the medical schools] that every night bodies were taken over, and he supposed they were from the Almshouse. About three weeks ago a body was found lying near the fence of the grounds, and it is supposed that the resurrectionists had been disturbed in their work.[109]

While the almshouse provided Philadelphia medical schools with a consistent supply of bodies for many years, that wasn't always the case. The *New York Times* reported in 1879 that, despite no law sanctioning it, Philadelphians mistakenly believed that the almshouse was a legal source of bodies throughout the institution's history.[110] It was a right based on custom rather than law, which meant it could be revoked at any time. When there was conflict between the Guardians and physicians, or when the almshouse cracked down and tried—but ultimately failed—to stop body snatching due to public pressure, there were significant disruptions for years. Physicians, students, and medical schools not associated with Blockley also had to find their own regular supply of bodies outside of the almshouse, primarily from cemeteries.

The almshouse's dead were exploited in other ways than just body snatching. In addition to dissection, physicians preserved specimens as teaching tools and for research so that they could directly observe the structure of parts of the human body. With the development of pathological anatomy in the 19th century, such collections were used to study causes and effects of disease on the body's organs and tissues.[111] An attempt was made to establish a museum in the almshouse in 1814, and resident physicians were required to prepare specimens of interest, such as "A corroded kidney" and a "fetal preparation showing the vessels peculiar to circulation."[112] Wet specimens were kept in a liquid solution, usually of alcohol, what one Blockley resident physician called a "sort of alcoholic immortality."[113]

In 1858, Chief Medical Officer Dr. Smith was rumored to be selling dead inmates. A member of the almshouse committee charged with investigating the incident noted that there was an expectation among the community for reform in care for the almshouse's dead before the incident. However, the committee reported that instead of selling bodies, Dr. Smith preserved two of them due to their medical interest, but they were stolen by a physician not associated with the almshouse. If not body snatching, it represented clear mismanagement. How was someone able to come in and walk out with two bodies? It wasn't until 1860 that a museum was actually established in the almshouse for pathological specimens, which in 1874 included 322 specimens: "Osseous [bone] 71; nervous 14; integumentary and connective tissue 4; digestive apparatus 71; respiratory 26; vascular 44; genito-urinary 70; unclassified tumors, 7; calculus [stone], concretions, etc., 7."[114] During a period when the museum fell into disrepair, some specimens went missing.

One of the most famous anatomical museums today is the Mütter Museum, a Philadelphia medical history museum that displays specimens collected in this era. Thomas Dent Mütter, educated at the University of Pennsylvania and chair of surgery at Jefferson Medical College, donated his personal collection of anatomical preparations to the College of Physicians of Philadelphia, the oldest medical society in the country, which runs the museum that opened in 1863. Mütter collected the specimens from a wide range of sources, including Blockley.

Caspar Wistar, who succeeded William Shippen Jr. as Penn's second professor of anatomy, founded the university's Anatomical Museum in 1809; some of the specimens came from the almshouse where he practiced.[115] The collection formed the basis of what would become today's Wistar Institute, which was built on land bought from Blockley.[116] Today the institute is famous for the "Wistar Rat," which was the first "standardized" animal, or strain of rat, to be widely used in medical research. Wistar's collection and the Mütter Museum were two of America's largest anatomy museums in the 19th century.[117] Some of the Wistar collection specimens were stolen by a curator in the mid-20th century.[118]

Human skeletons were also important teaching tools, and almshouse surgeon David Hayes Agnew once drew the ire of the Cochranville, Pennsylvania community he lived in for his unusual method of preparing bones for study. There were many methods to loosen flesh before carving it off, and none were pretty: using quicklime, boiling, or leaving a body

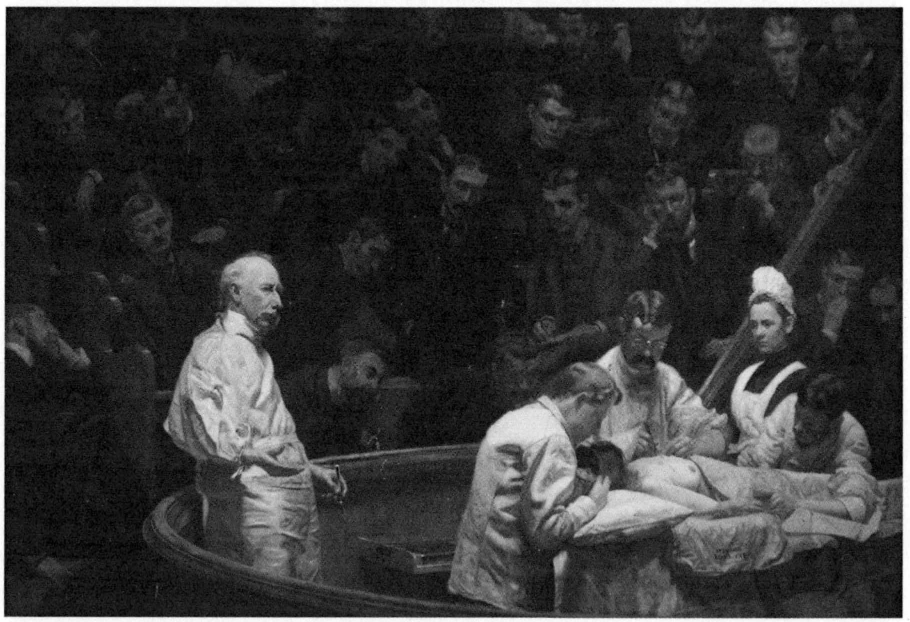

The Agnew Clinic, by Thomas Eakins (1889). David Hayes Agnew, left, holds a scalpel while performing an operation. (Wikimedia Commons)

submerged in water.[119] Agnew's method, which he used on bodies purchased from Philadelphia, was to place them in a nearby pond filled with eels that ate the flesh and left only bone behind. A local fisherman sold eels that came from the pond, which were very popular, "famed for their size and fatness," until one day he realized why.[120] A biographer of Agnew dryly noted that the discovery "did not increase the popularity of the young anatomist to any great extent."[121] It is not known if almshouse bodies were used to prepare skeletons, but it is hard to imagine that it never happened in the institution's long history.

Samuel George Morton, a resident physician in Blockley, collected and received human skulls from fellow physicians who practiced in the almshouse, some of which were from formerly enslaved Black Philadelphians.[122] Morton's collection of skulls, one of the largest in the world, was used to support the pseudoscientific idea that Black people were an inferior, separate human species, which was once taught in medical schools like the University of Pennsylvania. The skulls justified scientific racism, white supremacy, and slavery by claiming that differences between the skulls of Black and white people were evidence of differences in intelligence. Morton donated his collection of over 1,300 skulls to Philadelphia's Academy of Natural Sciences, where it was displayed for many years, but in 1966 the Penn Museum (formerly known as the University of Pennsylvania Museum of Archaeology and Anthropology) acquired the collection. The skulls were displayed in a classroom in the Penn Museum until it was put into storage in 2020 after protests by students.

In 1888 the "unclaimed" body of a 36-year-old Black woman named Harriet Cole, who died of tuberculosis in Philadelphia Hospital, was sent to Hahnemann Medical College (now Drexel University College of Medicine).[123] The anatomist Rufus B. Weaver did far more than simply dissect her: he extracted and mounted her nervous system for display, in the shape of a human body.[124] "Harriet," as the specimen became known, was the first complete dissection of the human cerebrospinal nervous system, the product of an enormous amount of painstaking work that became an important and widely influential tool for instruction and research.[125] It even won a blue ribbon at the 1893 World's Fair.[126]

While it was once believed that Cole donated her body for dissection, there is no evidence to support that claim. Today Harriet is on display as part of a medical history exhibit at Drexel University.

Almshouse inmates were also used for less educational purposes. In 1868 a 28-year-old Irish widow named Mary Lynch was admitted to Philadelphia Hospital for tuberculosis.[127] She died six months later from the wasting disease, and weighed only 60 pounds in the end.[128] Before her burial in the almshouse's graveyard, John Stockton Hough, a young Blockley resident physician who graduated from Penn, performed an autopsy on Lynch (an autopsy is made to determine a person's cause of death, while a dissection is made to study the structure of the human body). What Hough discovered inside her chest was truly horrifying: an estimated 8,000,000 cysts that teemed with *Trichinella spiralis*, a type of parasite known as the "pork worm." Lynch's death had been hastened by an act of kindness: her family brought her a ham and bologna sandwich that, unbeknownst to them, carried the food-borne parasite. In the article Hough published about the case, he wrote that Lynch was the first-known case of trichinosis in Philadelphia.

Hough did more than just autopsy Lynch before she was laid to rest: he also removed skin from her thigh and tanned it in a chamber pot in Blockley's basement, and nearly 20 years later bound three books about women's health using her skin.[129] We only know whose skin the book came from by a note Hough wrote in one of the books about Mary.[130] Anthropodermic bibliopegy, the practice of binding books in human skin, is rare, but with five such books the Mütter Museum has one of largest collections in the world, three of which are from Lynch.[131] One of the other books was also Hough's, made from the skin of a man who passed away in Philadelphia Hospital in 1869, who might have been named Thomas McCloskey, and the last was a copy of *An Elementary Treatise on Human Anatomy*, written by Penn's professor of anatomy, Joseph Leidy, who had his personal copy of his work bound in the skin of a Civil War soldier he likely treated.[132]

The University of Pennsylvania has one of Hough's skin-bound books. Other objects were also historically wrapped in human skin, such as purses used to hold surgical instruments; the Mütter Museum had a wallet purported to be made out of skin by a Philadelphia physician, which was later proven to be made of animal leather.[133] The Anthropodermic Book Project, which has developed a method to scientifically determine whether books are in fact made of human skin, has confirmed that out of the 32 books they have inspected, 18 of them were actually made out of human skin, and 14 were not.[134] The motivations of Hough and others who bound books in skin, which was largely performed by 19th-century physicians, is difficult to comprehend. If it was a form of commemoration, a tribute to honor their memory, it was certainly a strange way to show it. If anything, it reflected how physicians believed they could use the bodies of the poor in any way they saw fit, even for macabre personal book collections.

In 1882 an almshouse committee recommended separating Philadelphia Hospital from the almshouse, because "very few people are willing to go there for treatment, feeling that it involves being classed as a pauper, and it was recommended that the pauper element be placed elsewhere, leaving the Almshouse buildings for hospital purposes."[135] In 1902 Philadelphia Hospital became officially known as Philadelphia General Hospital, and in 1920 remaining inmates were removed from the almshouse to a facility in Holmesberg, and inmates with mental health issues were moved to Byberry, which suffered from similar problems as the almshouse, such as overcrowding and poor conditions.[136] Once only part of the almshouse, the hospital took over the entire institution, and as Philadelphia General Hospital became a site of not just care but medical advancement, it no longer carried the stigma it had in the past as the city's sole public hospital.

★ ★ ★

From its beginnings in the early 1730s, the almshouse provided care to the neediest Philadelphians, and was one of the earliest teaching hospitals. After the institution became Philadelphia General Hospital, it continued to do so, and for a time became one of the country's best public hospitals, which specialized in a number of areas, including ophthalmology and radiology.[137] It was the first hospital to provide radiology tests to diagnose cancer in 1921.[138] But in 1977, after almost two and a half centuries of providing medical care, Philadelphia General Hospital was shut down for good by Mayor Frank Rizzo, who cited the high costs to the city for the decision. Today Philadelphia is one the few major cities in the country to have no publicly funded general hospital.[139]

Almshouses were commonplace in mid-19th-century America, but gradually disappeared by the mid-20th century as they were replaced by social services.[140] Poor relief came full circle: instead of "indoor" relief, or institutionalizing the poor, "outdoor" relief in the form of Social Security became standard after Franklin D. Roosevelt signed the Social Security Act in 1935, although the system differed from traditional outdoor relief in that it was not freely given, but funded by payroll taxes, a system, of course, that has its own problems of funding and sustainability.

In 2002—a year after the bones of almost 450 people in Blockley's second graveyard were uncovered alongside the west bank of the Schuylkill River, during the construction of a parking garage—the University of Pennsylvania and the nearby Children's Hospital of Philadelphia (which was built on part of Blockley's former grounds) petitioned Philadelphia's Court of Common Pleas to rebury the bones in the nearby Woodlands Cemetery, a request that was approved.[141] The University of Pennsylvania's Civic Center Boulevard parking garage stands on what was Blockley's second graveyard. Today all that remains of Blockley almshouse is a fence that stands on Civic Center Boulevard.[142] In 2004 the bodies of three headless children were discovered in the Bettering House's second graveyard in Center City, also during construction.[143]

The Philadelphia Hospital was underfunded and overcrowded with inadequate facilities, but it provided a training ground for medical students and new doctors who were able to treat some of the city's most desperate, and made important medical advances. While a 21st-century archaeological study of Blockley's graveyards showed that Blockley physicians dissected any bodies they could get their hands on, the burden was disproportionately borne by almshouse residents, the most vulnerable members of society: the destitute, the sick and the terminally ill, the elderly, the widowed, children, and the mentally ill, among others.[144]

Medical care was certainly improved by what physicians learned in treating almshouse residents, benefits that also accrued to inmates themselves. Many generations of doctors learned how to treat and help others by practicing in the almshouse, and the research conducted there and published in medical journals undoubtedly contributed to medical progress. The almshouse also treated those whom no one else would, but it was an imperfect refuge, and one that did not always serve the residents' best interests. Blockley became the Philadelphia medical community's primary source of bodies in the 19th century, which directly led to Philadelphia's ascent as the country's center of medicine and medical education through the delegitimization of the poor's claims to proper burial.

A tangible legacy Blockley left behind were collections of specimens and other objects, such as books bound in human skin taken from almshouse residents, which are now the subject of debates that revolve around an important question: in an era before medical consent, can human remains obtained through body snatching or other means be ethically displayed in places like the Mütter Museum? While medical consent is a modern concept, virtually no one at the time would have willingly donated their bodies for dissection, let alone to have their organs displayed in perpetuity.

One approach to answering these thorny ethical questions is to listen to ancestral communities, to see how the community that was affected by this exploitation would like to commemorate the dead, such as through repatriation, or reburial. But if there is no one to speak for the dead, is there a way to respectfully display the remains for educational or research purposes? What does respectful treatment mean, and what would preserving the dignity of the dead in this context look like? Are we continuing this exploitation by displaying such specimens, or does the educational value outweigh other considerations? There are no easy answers, and the story of these collections didn't begin or end with the almshouse, but were part of a larger narrative of body snatching in Philadelphia and the United States.

Although the Guardians didn't always agree with physicians, the almshouse's long history of body snatching happened on their watch. The medical community was of course responsible for the rise of body snatching, but the almshouse's management also played a part, if only through their negligence, in allowing body snatching to flourish. Another reason why body snatching was so pervasive was something the public was unaware of: secret agreements that facilitated, and regulated, the exploitation of the almshouse's dead. When such agreements were in place, physicians didn't have to sneak into the cemetery at night to steal bodies. Instead, they picked them up, an arrangement that had the assent of even Philadelphia's mayor. The time of the "professional" resurrectionist was arriving, but for many years physicians didn't need their services when they had the support of the city in taking the dead for dissection.

CHAPTER 3

"The Philadelphia Method"

Secret Agreements and the Cadaver Trade

> At this moment in Philadelphia, we fortunately have a police, which is not disposed to interfere with us; but since the opening of our lectures, the town has been so uncommonly healthy, that I have not been able to obtain a fourth part of the subjects required for our dissecting rooms.
>
> —WILLIAM E. HORNER, PROFESSOR OF ANATOMY, UNIVERSITY OF PENNSYLVANIA, 1824[1]

On a cold morning in October 1846, residents of Philadelphia's Quince Street, in what we would call Center City today, made an alarming discovery: a dead body in an alley behind a newly opened medical school. The corpse was shrouded by a sack, except for its feet, which protruded from one end. The sight created "quite an excitement in the vicinity of the college," as the *Public Ledger* reported.[2] The strangeness of the situation only deepened when authorities determined what happened. The body belonged to a man who died in a local public institution over a week before, possibly the almshouse, but what looked like a body snatching gone wrong turned out to be something else entirely: an act of sabotage. The corpse was deliberately left in the alley to scandalize the college, which may have had its intended effect. Franklin Medical College was open for just three years before it closed its doors.[3]

Until Jefferson Medical College was established in 1824, the University of Pennsylvania was Philadelphia's sole medical school. More would follow. Some, like Franklin Medical College, came and went. Others, like Jefferson and Penn, still thrive today. The Woman's Medical College of Pennsylvania, the first medical school for women in the world, and Hahnemann Medical College, both founded in the mid-19th century, merged to become Drexel University's College of Medicine in 1993. Private anatomy schools also proliferated in the city to provide extracurricular dissections for medical students, such as the Philadelphia School of Anatomy, which operated from 1820 to 1875. We'll never know for sure who was responsible for the public spectacle on Quince Street, but if it wasn't an accident, it may have been a rival anatomist or medical school.

As medical education rapidly expanded in 19th-century Philadelphia, and America at large, so did competition for students, and an increasingly scarce commodity: bodies. It got ugly. According to Penn's medical faculty, a body was taken by force from the university in 1824, presumably one they had snatched, to a private anatomy school, after which students were used not just to study bodies but to protect them.[4] When they weren't coming to blows, anatomists bribed cemetery superintendents to secure exclusive rights to the dead. A solution was needed to end the free-for-all over the city's dead, to ensure an equitable distribution of the dead for dissection.

The primary source of "subjects" in 19th-century Philadelphia was the almshouse, not by chance, but in part by secret agreements that regulated the plunder of public burial grounds. In Philadelphia it was a conspiracy that went to the highest levels of the political establishment.[5] The dead deposited in the city's potter's fields, including the almshouse's, were systematically removed and delivered to medical schools without interference from the authorities. "Respectable" Philadelphians buried in churchyards were left undisturbed, and only the city's marginalized communities suffered the fate that all avoided if they could. Such arrangements were hidden from the public, but the truth eventually came out in public feuds and indiscreet private letters.

Bodies were also sold and shipped across the country on railroads, to and from Philadelphia, in the "cadaver trade." Body snatching no longer had borders, but the steady supply of "anatomical material" to Philadelphia's medical schools and around the country—and the secret agreements that facilitated it—were precarious. Feuds between physicians threatened to expose the secrets of the dissecting room to the public and risked the entire enterprise of anatomy education in the city.

★ ★ ★

When James Webster wrote, "I am about to engage for the first time in a mode of warfare I dislike," he wasn't referring to violence, but a war of words: a pamphlet.[6] Just as "flame wars" regularly erupt online today, "pamphlet wars" were waged in the past.[7] Thomas Paine's *Common Sense* was crucial in swinging public opinion on the side of independence from Great Britain when it was published in 1776. But while anyone can effortlessly share their opinions on the internet today, pamphlets first had to be typeset, printed, and distributed, so there was at least some time to reconsider an ill-advised message.

To the dismay of Philadelphia's anatomists, that didn't stop Webster. He published the innocuous-sounding *Facts Concerning Anatomical Instruction in Philadelphia* in 1832 to respond to accusations against his character. Its contents were explosive. Determined to defend his honor, consequences be damned, Webster wrote, "I regarded the *lex talionis* [an eye for an eye] as perfectly justifiable under the circumstances, and determined that if I must fall I would not come down singly, but bring those who would oppress me to the same level."[8] His supposed oppressor? The University of Pennsylvania's anatomy faculty.

Born in England in 1803, Webster's family moved to Philadelphia when he was young. He graduated from Penn with a degree in medicine in 1824, and two years later taught anatomy in a private anatomy school—the Philadelphia Anatomical Rooms (later known as the Philadelphia School of Anatomy)—located behind Penn's 9th Street campus, where he replaced the esteemed John Davidson Godman. Webster's classes were said to be "crowded, and he succeeded in imparting to his students the same enthusiasm which he himself felt in the study of his favorite science," although a history of the school noted that he was "not so polished and industrious as Godman."[9] Despite the school's closeness to Penn, they were not competitors. With its additional opportunities for dissection, the Philadelphia Anatomical Rooms supplemented a university education.[10] For much of the 19th century the standards of medical education were not particularly high, and the pathway to a medical career or to obtain a medical degree not as rigorous as today. Extracurricular dissections, and teaching hospitals like Philadelphia Hospital, were one way for students to gain hands-on surgical experience beyond the usual lectures and medical texts before they graduated to practicing on the living.

By 1830 something had changed in the relationship between the school and Penn, and an advertisement Webster placed for his series of courses was defensive:

> Dr. Webster deems it proper to state, that neither do his lectures nor dissecting establishment interfere with the regulations, time, or duties of the University [Penn]; Medical Students, in all Medical Institutions, are at liberty to pursue their dissecting studies under a private or public teacher, as they may please; it is thought advisable to mention these facts, the contrary having been stated.[11]

Whether Webster anticipated a fight or tried to start one is uncertain, but sparks soon flew regardless. In preparation for the lectures Webster contacted his usual supplier of bodies, "the agent," who assured him that he would receive his share on time. None came, but Webster noticed that Penn's demonstrator of anatomy, John P. Hopkinson, received his quota. Webster approached Penn's professor of anatomy, William E. Horner, who also served as the medical school's dean, about the discrepancy.

Webster and Horner had entered into an agreement two years before (in 1828) that divided the dead buried in Philadelphia's public burial grounds, "adopted as a code by which anatomists shall be governed."[12] The scope of the arrangement is unclear, but it encompassed at least Penn and multiple private anatomy schools. Its purpose was to "sustain the medical interests of Philadelphia, and to prevent the public scandal and excitement incident to the cultivation of anatomy," as it read.[13] In other words, it was designed to keep anatomists' dealings secret by heading off open conflict. As Penn's medical faculty described in a letter from 1824, groups of anatomists from different medical and private anatomy schools tried to steal bodies from the same cemetery the same night and got into fights, which drew attention to something that was normally conducted in secret.[14]

Anatomists in other states had similar arrangements. In 1885 Ohio anatomists agreed that whichever party made it to the graveyard first would not be interfered with, but it was a different story when it actually happened. One night a group of intoxicated physicians arrived at a cemetery where a body snatching was already in progress, and instead of backing down they started a fight. After losing they alerted the town that a body snatching was in progress, and the Western Reserve University Medical School's group had to run and leave the body behind, as physician Frederick C. Waite recalled.[15] Like in Ohio, agreements weren't always followed to the letter in Philadelphia either.

When Webster met with Horner, he expected an explanation but was instead given the runaround: Horner referred Webster to Hopkinson about the issue, and Hopkinson referred Webster to Horner. Finally, with his friend Francis S. Beattie, a fellow physician, Webster confronted Hopkinson and demanded the corpses he was owed as part of the arrangement, "peaceably if we could, forcibly if we must."[16] Hopkinson agreed that Webster would receive his allotment, but none came even after Webster's threat, while the deliveries to Penn, and their excuses, mounted. Webster claimed that Hopkinson told his class to "keep quiet a day or two gentleman—these [bodies] belong to Webster, but he cannot get them out!"[17] But Webster wasn't about to back down; his career was at stake. If he couldn't supply cadavers for his classes, he couldn't teach.

Backed into a corner, Webster escalated the conflict. He and his "professional friends" kept, in his words, a "strict observance…upon the operations of the agent."[18] This was a nice way of saying that Webster deployed the nuclear option: he somehow managed to stop the agent from delivering bodies to Penn or any other private anatomists for over a week, which stopped dissections in the affected schools. Horner and Hopkinson did not take this kindly, and Webster wrote in his pamphlet that they hired "ruffians" who were "well armed" to stop him.[19] It wouldn't be the first time anatomists came to blows over the dead in Philadelphia. But the threat of violence never materialized, and the blockade was successful: Horner seemingly relented. As before, Horner proceeded again to do nothing, and a series of increasingly indignant letters ensued. Their fight would then be one of words.

Webster believed Horner withheld bodies to put private anatomists like himself out of business, to maintain their monopoly on medical education in Philadelphia. There was some truth to this. Penn had prevented previous attempts to form a competing medical school in the city by lobbying the Pennsylvania legislature, until the university failed to stop the opening of Jefferson Medical College (technically, Jefferson College's charter was extended to include a medical school).[20] On the other side, Horner claimed Webster violated the agreement when he obtained bodies from cemeteries outside the Philadelphia public burial grounds specified in the agreement (in Lancaster, New Castle, and Easton). But a history of the Philadelphia Anatomical Rooms offered an explanation that made more sense than Webster's or Horner's: "at one time, when there was greater difficulty than usual in getting subjects,—a chronic ailment of dissecting-rooms,—he [Webster] sat up night after night, watching that neither the University nor any private room should obtain them till he was supplied, and gained his point."[21]

In other words, Horner kept Webster's share to make up for a shortage of bodies, not because Webster violated the agreement or to put him out of business. But quarrels between anatomists for cadavers were apparently so expected that a process for resolving conflict was built into the arrangement: arbitration. A panel of three—representatives of the affected parties and a chairman—considered the case and made the judgment that Horner was at fault in the dispute. Agreements or no, when bodies were scarce the competition became cutthroat. Bad blood over the affair persisted (physicians were a feuding bunch), and Webster published the pamphlet to address rumors of "dishonorable conduct" on his part during the disagreement.[22]

The impact of the pamphlet at the time is unknown. It wouldn't be surprising if no anatomists responded, because a protracted pamphlet war was in no one's interest. Whatever followed was probably done privately, out of view from most Philadelphians. While the pamphlet was published publicly, Webster was careful to redact the word "bodies" from it. Whenever the word was used he replaced it with dashes: "I was entitled of right to the two—[bodies]—and to as many until I supplied the same number of classes as my neighbors."[23] But it wasn't difficult to read behind the lines to understand what was really being said, and anatomists' secret dealings were out in the open for all to see.

Webster left Philadelphia in the mid-1830s for an anatomy position in New York's Geneva Medical College, and the Philadelphia Anatomical Rooms continued operating until 1875, when it finally closed its doors.[24] Horner continued to teach at Penn until his death in 1853. While the actual agreement is likely lost, a private letter by the man Webster originally replaced at the Philadelphia Anatomical Rooms, John D. Godman, revealed much more about what the arrangement might have contained, and how even the mayor of Philadelphia was involved in the trafficking of the city's dead.

When John D. Godman left Philadelphia in 1826 for a position at New York's Rutgers Medical College, he was one of the most advanced anatomists in the country.[25] But his tenure in New York, and his life, was short-lived. He soon resigned from his new position due to illness and returned to Philadelphia. In 1829, a year before his death at age 35 (and a year before Webster's dispute with Horner and Hopkinson), Godman wrote to John Collins Warren, professor of anatomy and surgery at Harvard Medical School, the medical school's first dean, and founder of the *New England Journal of Medicine*, one of the most prestigious medical journals today. In recognition of the sensitive nature of his letter, Godman ended it by writing, "All these statements, are of course secrets," which he hoped would help Warren "be successful in convincing your city authorities [in Boston] to view this matter aright."[26] With experience in both New York and Philadelphia, Godman was well positioned to explain how the system of supplying subjects worked in both cities, and which he preferred.

He started with New York. There were two pits in the public burial ground: one was for bodies that the cemetery's superintendent judged should receive respect, or were more likely to be claimed by friends, while the other was for everyone else—free and enslaved Black people, the poor, and other marginalized New Yorkers.[27] Anatomists were free to take the latter, so long as they notified the "keeper" when they planned to retrieve them at night so they could help conceal evidence of their evening incursion the next morning.

But Godman preferred Philadelphia's system to New York's. He called the "Philadelphia Method," or arrangement, "vastly superior." Describing how it worked, he wrote:

> The city appoints a superintendent to each of the public grounds at a very small salary. It is perfectly understood that his *business* is to give the anatomists every facility consistent with the most entire secrecy. He is allowed to profit thereby as much as may be; observing with strict justice to supply each applicant in his turn according to the nature of his claim, which is determined by the number in his class.[28]

Superintendents were incentivized to keep the proceedings quiet by taking the profits, and the number of bodies allocated to each anatomist depended on the size of their classes. Superintendents didn't need any convincing to do this dirty work; they were hired for it. Godman continued:

> These superintendents have their own servants and at certain hours of the night agreed upon between the city watch and themselves they are permitted to deliver the subjects to the anatomical establishments free from interruption. In case of misconduct or unfair dealing on the part of the superintendents, the anatomist makes complaint to the mayor of the city, who inquires into—and regulates the matter. In Philadelphia *all* the subjects buried in the two public grounds from the 1st Nov. till the first of April, can be had for dissection if required.[29]

When Webster referred to his supplier of bodies as "the agent," he may have been referring to the servants of superintendents. The dead were delivered to medical schools with impunity, with no opposition from the burial ground, city watch, police, or mayor, who intervened if there were any troubles. Body snatching, an enterprise usually fraught with risk, became a function of the city. Unlike New York, *all* bodies buried in Philadelphia's public burial grounds were open for the taking. None apparently deserved the respect of a proper burial.

> The Philadelphia method is decidedly the most advantageous to all parties. It is the interest of the keeper to manage every thing with the utmost caution, and therefore there is never the slightest danger from popular tumult, as nothing can ever be seen by passers, that would lead to suspicion, and few persons in the city have the slightest idea of the manner in which the schools are supplied or even that they are supplied. A very strict watch is kept over the grounds, by the persons employed by the keeper, but it is to prevent private adventurers from

> robbing *him*—not to prevent them from emptying the pits...a popular disturbance or robbery of a private burial ground is unknown, notwithstanding from 12 to 20 subjects are weekly consumed during the dissecting season.[30]

The Philadelphia arrangement maintained secrecy surrounding how the city's medical schools were supplied with subjects, and prevented body snatching in private cemeteries, which drew unwanted attention. A watch was kept not to ensure bodies wouldn't be taken, but to ensure that they were taken by the right parties. While there are a number of possible public burial grounds that the letter could have been referring to, one of them may have been the Bettering House's graveyard, as the almshouse was known then. It's uncertain if the agreement Godman wrote about was the same as Webster and Horner's. They struck their arrangement in 1828, Godman wrote his letter to Warren in 1829, and the Webster and Horner conflict erupted in 1830, so the timing is right. If so, it meant that when there were not enough bodies the agent could be bribed or controlled, despite measures like arbitration in place to prevent it—if not the intervention of the mayor himself—and that anatomists could be their own worst enemies. Regardless of whether it was the same agreement, Godman's letter provided rare insight into how they worked in practice.

Godman's letter raised questions with answers that are likely lost to history. How did such arrangements come about? What other incidents were there that led to an agreement like Webster and Horner's? How long were they in place? There were far too many public body-snatching scandals from private burial grounds for them to have always been in place. Why were the authorities willing to go along with it? The medical community was a politically influential group that held sway, but the authorization of the wholesale body snatching of public cemeteries was a big ask, to say the least. Philadelphia's growing dominance in the medical field, and its economic importance for the city, may have played a role.

What we do know is that such arrangements were not confined to the borders of Philadelphia or other states with medical schools. Before Warren corresponded with Godman about how body procurement worked in Philadelphia and New York, he wrote to Horner seeking bodies. In 1824 Horner replied:

> The scarcity is felt with still greater severity, in consequence of the influx of students, exceeding that of any former year. I now count on my matriculation list, four hundred and seventy five students, nearly two hundred of whom are in my dissecting class. While this scarcity continues, I am left in an incessant state of anxiety, by the eagerness of the new students to commence operations, and thus disappointment at postponement. Anatomically speaking when the times become more propitious, I shall then be able to turn my attention to the wants of friends. I have no expectation of being free on this point at the time [December] mentioned by you.[31]

Such scarcity helps explain why Horner was willing to go as far as he did in his conflict with Webster six years later. Horner was forced to source bodies from New York when there was a shortage in Philadelphia; at other times it was New York physicians who were scouring Philadelphia for bodies.[32] Philadelphia wasn't the only source of bodies for Philadelphia-based anatomists, and the same was true in other states. A little-known part of the history of body snatching is that corpses were imported and exported across the United States.

Body snatching became a problem across the country in cemeteries near medical schools—starting in Philadelphia—but for a time it was largely a local affair, although medical schools tried to convince the public otherwise. When a body was snatched from St. Mary's Church in Philadelphia in 1841, the *Public Ledger* reported, "Lest injustice should be done, by imputing this outrage to innocent parties, we are authorized to say that it was not known of, or sanctioned by the faculty of either of the medical schools in this city [Penn or Jefferson]."[33] Newspapers would blame individual body snatchers, or medical students from distant cities, when a local medical school was a much more likely culprit.[34] But with the rise of the inter-state trade in cadavers, Philadelphians could have been dissected in any state where their transportation there was feasible.

The development of one technology changed body snatching forever: railroads. Of all the transformative effects of railroads on American life—where people lived, how they traveled, and even their sense of time with the standardization of time zones—few could have imagined that they would be used for the long-distance trade in the dead.[35] Bodies were shipped from north to south, and south to north, including enslaved Black people, and everywhere in between, with a size and scope few realized at the time or even today. Medical schools could now be supplied from anywhere in the country, a trade that was sometimes even facilitated by deals with railroad companies to convey the dead.

★ ★ ★

One frigid night in December 1873, Washington, D.C., police officers noticed a horse and buggy sitting idle near Washington Circle.[36] Its only occupant was a woman named Margaret Harrison, and when the officers approached her, she explained that her husband was working nearby. Their suspicions raised, the police decided to keep watch. After midnight two men approached the buggy with shovels caked with dirt, but neither was Harrison's husband. They were her partners in crime: George Christian, graduate of a local medical school and a clerk in the Surgeon General's office, and his assistant Charles Green. The men disinterred the dead, while Harrison posed as a mourner at funerals to locate their victims.

All three body snatchers were said to have been intoxicated to some degree. Christian was "a man of medium build, athletic, strong-muscled, of great endurance, and a good worker in the cause [of body snatching]; his hair and beard were black...His frequent raids and his sullenness when drinking were the causes of his undoing."[37] When the officers arrested the trio of body snatchers there was no body in the buggy, but a bag was discovered in the nearby Holmead's Burying Ground. The bag contained the body of Thomas Fletcher, a Black man buried the previous day, which was "doubled up in order to get it into the sack, with the head and the hands at the mouth of the same," a local newspaper reported.[38] Why they left the body behind is unknown. Christian refused to answer any questions, and with no law on the books at the time for body snatching, the trio were charged with "Carrying concealed weapons, disorderly conduct, suspicious character, and every imaginable thing."[39] When the officers searched Christian they found a loaded revolver, a membership card for the Young Men's Christian Association, and most significantly, a diary and letters that implicated him in a body-snatching ring that extended well beyond the nation's capital. Why Christian thought it would be a good idea to carry around a record of his criminal activities is anyone's guess.

Christian was a new kind of body snatcher—"the dealer in human bodies, who, procuring corpses, either by theft or by corruption, is able to distribute them at a high rate of payment to colleges throughout the country," as a contemporary Boston physician put it.[40] To use historian Daina Ramey Berry's term, Christian was a part of the "domestic cadaver trade," or "cadaver trade" for short, a decentralized network of medical schools and body snatchers that sold, bought, and transported cadavers with varying levels of organization and sophistication. Christian supplied Washington medical schools and shipped bodies to Virginia, Michigan, and Ohio, and likely other states as well.

Bodies were transported by resurrectionists like Christian in many ways, as a medical lecturer of the time recounted:

> The means of high medical education are accessible in many country institutions. Every intelligent man of the large cities…knows that the *materiel* [cadavers] of Anatomy is abundant and can be transported any where and every where—that Railroads, and Steamboats, and Transportation Lines, and Expresses, and the like, make the movement of the *materiel*…a matter of the least difficulty.[41]

But before modern embalming methods, the distance bodies could travel for dissection was limited, and speed was essential to the work of body snatchers. A putrefied body had limited usefulness for dissection, and if it was accepted for sale at all, it wouldn't fetch a good price. The cold acted as a natural preservative, which was why medical schools held sessions in the colder months, but it was a losing battle with nature; refrigeration technology was still in its infancy in the era of the body snatchers. Some were shipped from New York to what is now Harvard Medical School, and to Vermont in barrels labeled as food, transported by boat and wagon.[42]

Body snatchers used any transportation technology available to them, but railroads speeded the delivery of cadavers considerably, which made shipping them long distances more practical. Bodies were often shipped in barrels filled with a liquid, such as alcohol, which preserved and masked the smell of corpses in transit. The *Boston Medical and Surgical Journal* touted the preservative properties of alcohol in an 1835 article:

> To nine gallons of common New England rum, or whiskey, add an equal quantity of water—the whole being sufficient for covering an adult subject in a suitably constructed vessel. We have kept one or two, in this way, an entire year, and found them in most perfect condition for demonstration at the expiration of that time.[43]

Stories abound that upon delivery the barrel's alcohol was not wasted but sold by faculty to medical students who, knowingly or (probably) unknowingly, drank the "rotgut" whiskey.[44] Some say that the term "stiff" drink had its origins in this distasteful side business, but there is little historical evidence to support it. Still, some certainly imbibed the whiskey used in the preservation of the dead for medical education. A history of the Philadelphia Anatomical Rooms claimed that its

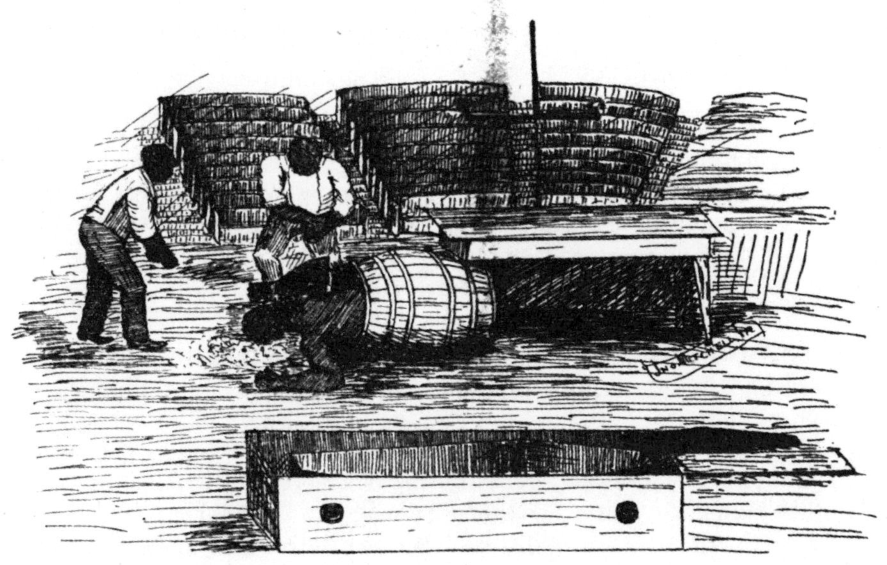

The person rolling up his sleeves represents Chris Baker; the other Funeral Director W. S. Selden, and the man partly in the barrel is Solomon Marable. In the rear are the empty benches usually occupied by students when the dissecting of a body is taking place. The Medical College of Virginia, corner of College and Marshall Sts., Richmond, Va., is the place.

A body delivered by barrel to the Medical College of Virginia in 1896. (Library of Congress)

janitor died from drinking specimen alcohol.[45] In 1865 a Rhode Island newspaper reported that a barrel of whiskey was stolen from a train, and the thieves realized only after they started drinking from it that a body was stored inside.[46]

Other methods of embalming at the time could be dangerous to those that administered them, such as arsenic, a danger that was well understood at the time. When Godman ran the Philadelphia Anatomical Rooms, "his janitor, from a scratch on his thumb nearly lost his life, and Dr. Godman himself was poisoned three times, once so severely that his arm was useless for some weeks…he made the great improvement of using whisky—an impure form of alcohol—for injection."[47] While unhealthy for the living, alcohol was effective in keeping the dead fresh. A barrel used for transporting bodies is currently on display in Davidge Hall at the College of Medicine of Maryland.

Corpses were also shipped in boxes, as Christian described in a letter he received from a Michigan physician that was published in newspapers after his arrest:

> Boxes have come, or rather barrels. Do not send barrels; they always get the heads knocked in, and excites suspicion if they do not, as the subjects shake about so. The best way to pack is in a tight box three feet by two, or near that dimension, the subject having legs and thighs flexed and head resting on chest. Sawdust packed about prevent odor and the subject from shaking about in the box. Two can be put in a single box a little larger than the one I describe.[48]

A letter Christian received from a Virginia physician, which was also made public, included a typical order for bodies:

> Please send me at once two subjects of merchantable quality and securely barreled. I have had infinite trouble in consequence of a bloody liquid escaping from one of the barrels last winter. Send them by freight to Dr. J.S. Davis, University of Va., and notify me by mail that you have sent them…P.S.—If the arrangement works well I will get from you chiefly.[49]

Christian had a number of associates, a colorful cast of characters that showed how just about anyone could be a body snatcher:

- a woman named "Workhouse" Kate;
- Percy Brown, "a big fellow, a good fighter, and of a very ugly disposition when he was drinking";

- Maude Pratt, who was either Percy's sister or common law wife ("it was never known which"), who "was a very devil; she married a disreputable dentist just about the time he [Percy] was dying";
- and a "negro preacher; he taught salvation and repentance to the limit on Sundays, buried the dead of his congregation; but the strain on his nervous system was so great that he was compelled to let off steam by stealing the bodies he so faithfully buried."[50]

A history of body snatching written by a D.C. physician also claimed that one of the people who worked for Christian was a ward physician, and the "death rate of that ward soared very high for the good of the cause."[51] Christian and his partners in crime had a "big and profitable business" that they originally ran out of a shack, but then moved to a local medical school:

> Christian would inject and pack the bodies in whiskey barrels at the college, roll these barrels up in front of the Army Medical Museum, where the express company would call for them; Christian was always on hand to pay charges and direct the shipments; in this way the company did not suspect the fraud. The price of bodies fluctuated with the demand and the weather. When the demand was great it was a common thing to charge one hundred dollars for a good subject; when the market became glutted the average price was forty dollars. Quite a number of Demonstrators paid a hundred dollars. Shipments were mostly to the South.[52]

All costs were accounted for and paid by the recipient, including bodies, barrels, whiskey, or if shipping in boxes, the packing material, and of course the labor. Body snatchers assumed the risk but not the cost of transporting bodies. The best methods for transporting bodies were learned through trial and error, and if caught, much was at stake: not just what was probably an expensive order of bodies, but the viability of entire transportation routes. Just as cemeteries were on high alert after a body snatching, so were railroads if a body was found in transit.

But the dead didn't always make it to their destination, or even on the train. An Iowa medical student named A. Mackey was arrested for receiving snatched bodies shipped by barrel on the Chicago, Rock Island and Pacific Railroad. Inside the barrel labelled "pickled pork," "The remains were in a shocking condition, having been placed in the barrel without any protection, and been begrimed and disfigured from jostling about in handling."[53] In 1845 a box shipped to an Ohio physician was opened due to the horrible smell emanating from it; the authorities found the bodies of a woman and child inside.[54] The infamous Cincinnati body-snatcher William Cunningham was caught trying to ship a body in a box marked "Glass with care" to a Kansas-based doctor.[55]

In Atlanta, Georgia, a package shipped to Arch Avery, a druggist, was accidently received by B. F. Avery, a businessman, who had the barrel labeled "kerosene" opened and discovered two bodies packed inside with charcoal.[56] In 1896 an employee of the United States Express Co. opened a box mistakenly labeled with two addresses—a box that had been reused—to see if he could glean any more information. When he placed his hand inside he was, to say the least, surprised to find a foot in his grasp.[57] There was one way to avoid such unfortunate mix-ups, and to reduce the risk of shipping bodies: make deals with railroads.

One known agreement was between John Staige Davis, one of Christian's customers, and the Virginia Central Railroad. After he graduated from the University of Virginia, Davis studied medicine in Philadelphia—likely in the almshouse—one of many Southern medical students who traveled north to learn in the center of American medicine. Southern students attended Penn or Jefferson and made up a surprisingly large amount of enrollment; three out of every five Penn students were Southern from 1831 to 1840.[58] Davis returned to teach anatomy in his *alma mater* in the mid-1840s, and what we know about Davis's dealings is thanks to the letters he kept, which provide unprecedented insight into the unenviable job of securing bodies for anatomy classes. Lewis W. Minor, a physician from Norfolk, wrote to Davis about the letters they exchanged: "I pray you to destroy them, for truly they have not even a respectable appearance."[59] Luckily for us he didn't.

Davis ran a complex operation, but one that didn't always run smoothly. The university set aside funds for Davis to purchase corpses, and he negotiated terms and made contracts with body snatchers, often through intermediaries. The bodies were shipped to Davis from the Virginia Central Railroad depot using a fake name so it couldn't be traced. But when a barrel en route to Davis—labeled "McIntire

Charlottesville"—was intercepted by an unsuspecting train station agent in 1850, they were forced to change it for the shipments that followed: "Of course all barrels boxes &c. large enough to contain your favorite article of trade, and addressed as above, will in future be closely scrutinized."[60] Davis's frustrations with the body snatcher who shipped the barrel came to a boil after the incident, and he resolved to withhold payment until *after* he received the bodies, and his intermediary ordered the body snatcher to put the date of the body's burial and shipment on the barrel.[61]

Davis experienced similar frustrations when he worked with other shifty body snatchers, but in 1851 he made a deal with Hampden-Sydney College medical school to end competition for bodies in Richmond, Virginia's capital. In exchange for Davis no longer employing a resurrectionist in Richmond, Hampden-Sydney would instead handle obtaining bodies and divide them up between both schools and deliver Davis's share by rail; Davis was free to source additional bodies outside of Richmond.[62] Cooperation, not competition, ensured a regular supply of bodies for all parties. Davis also struck up a deal with the Virginia Central Railroad later in 1851 to ensure the safe passage of the bodies, not by bribing a low-level railroad employee, but by making an agreement directly with Edmund Fontaine, the president of the railroad.

In private letters they haggled over the particulars. Bodies couldn't be shipped in baggage cars, and certainly not in passenger cars, only by freight, and in a car specifically for that purpose.[63] They discussed when and how bodies should be dropped off at the depot.[64] Price was a problem: the railroad agent kept raising rates for shipping bodies, and Davis didn't have much other choice but to pay.[65] Presumably, it was the money that led the railroad to enter into an agreement with Davis in the first place, but it was a small price for him to pay to ensure the safe passage of his sensitive cargo.

Sometimes there were too few bodies: "Richmond is so distressingly healthy at this time," an intermediary wrote to Davis to explain why there was a shortage of bodies, but at other times there were too many: "the Dissecting Room being previously crowded—Indeed, several of the subjects are still unpacked...ask Dr. Howard to communicate with the Resurrectionist again without the delay, & give him peremptory orders to stop, until further notice," Davis wrote.[66] But one medical school's scarcity was another school's surplus, and as in Virginia, Southern medical schools supplied each other: Alabama's oldest medical school, the Graefenberg Medical Institute, imported bodies from other parts of the state and New Orleans in molasses barrels.[67] A body snatcher in Tennessee shipped bodies in boxes labeled "fish" or "fur" to Atlanta, Georgia, as well as Ohio.[68] There were times of abundance and scarcity, but the cadaver trade helped close the gap and ensured more consistent access to the dead for medical education.

Baltimore, with its proximity to the Baltimore and Ohio Railroad (America's first common carrier) was known as the "resurrection city," a hub of the cadaver trade that supplied medical schools on the East Coast.[69] In 1836 Jefferson Medical College's demonstrator of anatomy purchased bodies through an intermediary in Baltimore.[70] Midwest and New England medical schools sourced their bodies from Maryland, a temperate zone, when the ground in their regions were too frozen to dig.[71] In response to a request for bodies, a Baltimore physician wrote to one based in Maine that they had no problems getting bodies, and that they could send them out of state.[72]

In the North and South, many if not most of the victims of body snatching, and those shipped in the cadaver trade, were likely Black. Daina Ramey Berry coined the term "domestic cadaver trade" to highlight its parallels with the slave trade, how enslaved people were bought and sold in life and death. Before the Civil War the primary source of subjects were enslaved Black people, who were also used to prepare anatomical specimens for Southern anatomical museums or personal collections, in part because, while medical schools in urban areas like Philadelphia were able to obtain bodies from institutions like almshouses, hospitals, and prisons, such options were not available in the rural South.[73] However, the bodies of enslaved Black people were easier to appropriate in the South than free Black people or other marginalized groups in Northern states. Enslavers could profit off the bodies of people they enslaved even after their death, and white Southerners had fewer qualms about the dissection of human beings they considered chattel.

Still, the demand for bodies was high and there were not always enough to supply medical schools.

Davis was also an enslaver who purchased Black people while they were alive, and after their death for dissection. The bodies of enslaved people were shipped from the South to the North to supply medical schools like the University of Pennsylvania, and from the North to the South.[74] When detected, the police didn't pay the trade much mind, according to James Silk Buckingham, a British man who traveled America in the 1830s:

> It had been discovered, that of late, it was a common practice in New York, to ship off the bodies of dead negroes, male and female, for various ports, but especially the south, to the medical students, for dissection... Yesterday morning it was discovered that a barrel, which had been put into the office of the Charleston packet line...for the purpose of being shipped to Charleston, contained the bodies of two dead negroes...The cask and contents were sent up to the police office, and placed in the dead-house for the Coroner's inspection...The verdict of the inquest, subsequently given...was, that the negroes had died of disease; but no further inquiry appears to have been made into the matter, as if it were altogether beneath the notice of the white men to trace out these traders in the dead bodies of the blacks.[75]

When Harriet Martineau, a British author, visited Maryland in 1835, she noted that "In Baltimore the bodies of coloured people exclusively are taken for dissection, 'because the whites do not like it, and the coloured people cannot resist.'"[76] Black cemeteries were the most vulnerable, in Maryland and other states, which was why they were targeted the most frequently.

The Civil War of course disrupted medical education north and south, and physicians like Davis treated wounded soldiers, and if they had the time also dissected the plentiful bodies available to them in the deadliest war in American history. The war had a transformative effect on medicine, especially in the field of surgery. Amputation was the most common surgical procedure, and given the sheer number performed during the bloody war, important advances were made in fields such as plastic surgery and prosthetics. While anesthesia was invented before the Civil War, in the 1840s—John Collins Warren, who wrote to Godman about body procurement in Philadelphia and New York, carried out the first successful public demonstration of surgery with a patient under anesthetic (using ether) in 1846 with the dentist William T. G. Morton—its widespread use during the war revolutionized the practice of surgery. Instead of operations being a test of the speed and strength of the surgeon, as a screaming patient experienced an unimaginable amount of pain, operations could be conducted deliberatively, and more carefully, which led to the ability to carry out more complex procedures, and to save more lives.

After the North won the war and the institution of slavery was abolished, the bodies of Black people were dissected and shipped across the country in the cadaver trade as they had been before. From 1880 until the end of the century, one New England medical school received two shipments of 12 Black people from the South each session, in barrels labeled "turpentine."[77]

After the Civil War, the threat of body snatching was also used to deter Black people in the South who, in search of economic opportunity—and to flee racial segregation and violence—migrated north, a loss of labor that threatened the Southern economy. One rumor spread by Southern landowners in an attempt to capitalize on the fear of body snatching to control Black people, was that medical men would ride through Black neighborhoods and abduct, murder, and take their bodies to experiment on them.[78] They went by many names: the "night doctors" or "night riders"—so called because they only struck in the evening—the "needle men" for the implement they used to subdue their victims, or the "black bottle men" who administered lethal medicine.

The story of the night doctors was effective because it had an element of truth: Black people were targeted by physicians for body snatching, but they generally didn't stoop to murder for medical education. Southerners reinforced these rumors by donning white gowns and riding through Black neighborhoods pretending to be night doctors.[79] Black oral histories provided the clearest evidence of the prevalence of such rumors and the fear they instilled, and showed that they were distinct from the Ku Klux Klan, but they were sometimes referred to as "Ku Klux doctors" due to their similarity.[80] Even as late as 1954, the night doctor was a boogeyman of children in Southern states, invoked by parents to scare their kids straight.[81] While the Tuskegee syphilis study, conducted between 1932 and 1972, is perhaps the most infamous case—in which participants who had the disease were left untreated to observe its effects on the body, despite the availability of penicillin to treat it—medical experimentation on Black people has a much longer history, which helps explain the persistence of the myth.

Aside from Davis and Christian, there were many other participants in the cadaver trade. A group of body snatchers led by Rufus Cantrell, "The King of Ghouls," operated in many states, including Indianapolis, Indiana, where he was caught shipping bodies to Ann Arbor and Detroit in Michigan.[82] In Ohio Charles Morton, an alias for Henri Le Caron, was also caught in 1878 shipping bodies to Michigan; his associates continued the operation after his arrest.[83] William Jansen, a body snatcher who operated in many states, but was most closely associated with Washington, D.C., was said to have supplied medical schools, "East, West, and South. Last winter, when bodies were said to be unusually scarce, he is reported as having shipped 25 barrels, each containing a doubled up body, from Washington to [Baltimore]…these bodies are said to have been shipped here by rail."[84]

Davis continued teaching at the University of Virginia until his death in 1885 from pneumonia.[85] After Christian, the D.C. body snatcher, was arrested he was sentenced to a year in jail. But in a head-spinning turn of events the medical community intervened, including faculty from two local medical schools, and by their recommendation and others his crimes were pardoned by President Ulysses S. Grant.[86] Having powerful friends kept many body snatchers like Christian out of jail. But that wasn't the end of Christian's story. Instead of reforming his ways, in 1875 he was caught shipping bodies from the Baltimore and Ohio depot.[87] He was arrested but managed to escape police custody, until he was caught in Baltimore, but not for long: he managed to escape *again*, and was never recaptured. On his deathbed in Philadelphia, a newspaper reported that Christian "piteously besought the woman he had lived with for a number of years not to let his remains fall into the hands of the medical fraternity. His dying request was that his body lie in a vault until decomposition had rendered it unfit for the dissecting table."[88]

Christian desperately wanted to avoid the fate that he had assured for so many others.

★ ★ ★

In the early 1820s a group of boys were playing in Southwark, Philadelphia, when they noticed a house with its door open.[89] Curiosity got the better of them and they stepped inside, but instantly regretted it: they came upon a corpse with a head that had been dissected. The boys ran and spread word of murder, and a mob converged on the house. The anatomist—who fled the scene—rented the house to perform dissections but failed to fully shut the front door that day. Penn's medical faculty warned the university's trustees that if Philadelphia's mayor had not been a strong supporter of science, the incident may have ended anatomy education in the city for a time.[90]

As the number of medical schools and private anatomy schools grew exponentially in the 19th century, a new mechanism was needed to prevent the public exposure of the secretive world of anatomy education. Medical schools, private anatomy schools, and operations like the one in Southwark that could hardly be called a "school" at all, fought for access to Philadelphia's dead. Secret agreements did not always calm the chaos of competition between anatomists, but while they were in effect they helped regulate the distribution of the dead in cities like Philadelphia and New York.

These arrangements were not just between individual anatomists and medical schools but involved local governments as well. Such grave dealings also extended not only within but between states, thanks to railroads, which revolutionized transportation of people, goods, and—unexpectedly—the dead, which made the country-wide trade in bodies possible, limited only by where the train lines ended. In Virginia at least, deals were even made with railroads to facilitate the transportation of bodies within the state. Like body snatching generally, the majority of victims were from marginalized groups, primarily enslaved or free Black people.

When such agreements broke down, or when bodies were not plentiful or were inaccessible in almshouses or other public institutions, the services of the "professional" body snatchers became invaluable. Who were the body snatchers? How did body snatching in Philadelphia and other cites work, and how exactly did they remove bodies from cemeteries? While the midnight raids of the body snatchers were very real, how they were understood was shaped not only by what they did, but by how they were represented in popular culture: newspapers, art, books, and even film. The era of the body snatchers, a time when physicians turned to the services of professionals to take the dead by force, was a strange, fascinating time when no cemetery in Philadelphia, or any other state, was safe from the demands of medical education. Like medicine, body snatching would become an industry, one that met the medical community's seemingly insatiable demand for bodies.

CHAPTER 4

Body Snatching

Myth and Reality

> I shall not tell how to properly snatch a body, as it might end disastrously for some of the younger men, and then again "lead us not into temptation."
>
> —FRANK BAKER, 1916[1]

One night in March 1859 the revelries of an Albany, New York "porter-house" were cut short by a cry for help.[2] The establishment's inhabitants were startled, not just by the sound that rang out shortly after midnight, but where it came from: a nearby cemetery. A half-dozen men put down their drinks and ran toward the wailing. Nothing could have prepared them for what they discovered as they approached one of the graves: a half-buried man, trapped in the earth, holding a corpse in his arms (featured on the cover of this book).

The man, named Bellew, had unearthed the grave, opened the coffin, and pulled out the corpse inside, but as the body snatcher handed it over to Johnson, his companion in crime, the grave caved in on itself. Johnson fled the scene and left his accomplice almost buried alive. The 15 dollars the physician promised them must not have been enough incentive to help his accomplice; there was no honor among thieves. The history of body snatching is shrouded in secrecy, and for good reason: a successful body snatching is one you don't know about. If you do, something went wrong. There was no manual for body snatching: it was a dark art, not a science.

Who were the body snatchers? They were widely believed to be "coarse and ignorant men, who had no scruples of conscience and were ready to undertake any job that promised to pay well," as a New York newspaper described practitioners of the trade in 1868.[3] How body snatchers were depicted in newspapers was similar to how they were described in literature. The 1846 novel *Marietta, Or the Two Students: A Tale of The Dissecting Room and "Body Snatchers"* depicted one body snatcher in harrowing terms:

> [He had a] ghastly visage—such a hollow corpse-like cheek—such a thin, sharp nose—such deeply sunken eyes—such a grim deformity for a mouth, whose lips hug closely the toothless gums, and such a frightful distance from the nether lip to the apex of the chin...did you ever gaze upon such a low, horribly wrinkled forehead, or greyer and more closely matted locks than his?[4]

Their real-life counterparts were men like William Cunningham, an Irish immigrant who supplied Cincinnati, Ohio's medical colleges with cadavers between 1855 and 1871.[5] "Old Cunny" was said to be a "big, raw-boned individual, with muscles like Hercules, and a protruding lower jaw, a ghoul by vocation, a drunkard by habit and a coward by nature."[6] His wife was also quite the character, "a bony, brawny, square-jawed Irish woman, with a mouth like an alligator. Both had a tremendous appetite for whiskey."[7] During the day Cunningham transported goods as a drayman, but at night he used his wagon for more nefarious purposes. Larger-than-life stories circulated around "The Prince of Ghouls." He was a boogeyman: parents would tell their misbehaving children stories about Cunningham.[8] According to a doctor he did business with:

> Usually he [Cunningham] took the body to town in a buggy. One night I met Cunny driving into town. There was a corpse sitting in the buggy on the seat beside him. The corpse was dressed up in an old coat, vest and hat. Cunny held the reins in his right hand while he steadied the corpse with his left arm around the waist of his silent companion. Every now and then the upper part of the corpse gravitated forward and downward. Whenever people passed, Cunny would slap his inoffensive partner in the face and say to him: "Sit up! This is the last time I am going to take you home when you get drunk. The idea of a man with a family disgracing himself in this way!" With such words and a few picturesque phrases by way of emphasis and rhetorical decoration, Cunny kept people from guessing the truth.[9]

Cunningham's shamelessness in the pursuit of body snatching, or more accurately, the pursuit of money, knew no bounds. He could also be cruel: once, after medical students played a joke on him, he delivered a body of a person who died of smallpox, which then spread among the students.[10] He was arrested multiple times for body snatching, but also got into trouble for his drinking, as an 1870 newspaper reported: "He first fired his brain with whisky then fired off an enormous revolver on Central Avenue."[11] Before "Old Man Dead" died in 1871 due to heart disease, he sold his body to the Medical College of Ohio where his skeleton was displayed in the college's museum; his wife managed to get five more dollars from the college for his corpse.[12] Cunningham clearly had no reservations about meeting the fate he meted out to so many others. His wife later joined a group of body snatchers.[13]

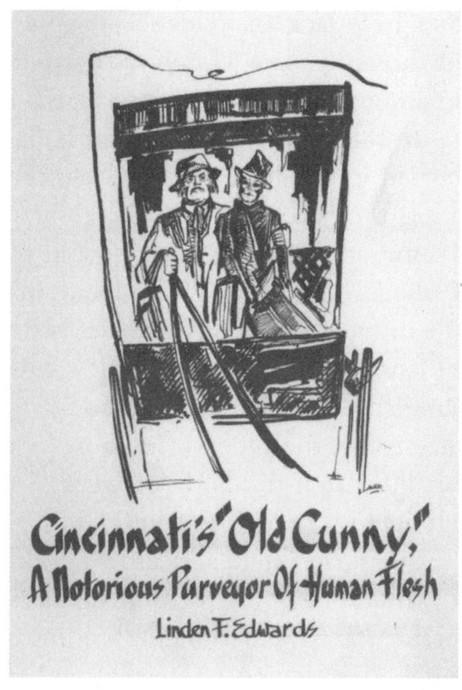

William Cunningham, an infamous 19th-century Ohio resurrectionist, props up the body he snatched. (Project Gutenberg)

William M. Jansen studied medicine in his native country of Denmark, but after he immigrated to the United States he turned to body snatching to fund his drinking problem.[14] The "Resurrectionist King," also known as Vigo Jansen Ross, was described as "bold, boastful, and revengeful."[15] When a reporter asked Jansen why he became a body snatcher, he replied, "it pays better than anything else that I know of."[16] He was active first in Baltimore. In 1880 a young woman named Jennie Smith died there. In one account it was the woman's mother who noticed something her daughter had been buried with atop the grave that caused the discovery of Jansen's crime.[17] In another account, the girl's aunt had a dream that Jennie's body had been stolen, and family and friends remembered that a stranger who attended the funeral had acted oddly, which led to the reopening of her empty grave and Jansen's arrest.[18] After he was let go due to a lack of evidence, he moved to Washington, D.C., the city he became most closely associated with, and where he famously, or infamously, stole a body twice.

In 1883 Charles Shaw was hanged for the murder of his sister and buried in the local potter's field, but not particularly deep.[19] Not long after, the "King of Ghouls" resurrected him in broad daylight in just 10 minutes. Jansen's assistant sold Shaw's body to Georgetown Medical College, but there was a problem. In some accounts the assistant pocketed the money, while in others Georgetown's medical students paid only half of Jansen's asking price. What happened next was not in dispute: Jansen stole the body back from the college to sell it a second time, but was arrested in the process. In court he told the judge, "Why, your honor, I would snatch the body of George Washington, could I but get to it."[20] He spent a year in prison, and Shaw was reburied in the potter's field.

Jansen later held a "lecture" on his ghoulish profession at the Theatre Comique in D.C. To calm his nerves he drank before and during the performance, but became too intoxicated to deliver it.[21] Heckled and laughed at, Jansen proceeded with a reenactment of a resurrection, but that didn't go any better: beneath a pile of dirt was a trap door, but when he tried to pull the "deceased" out of the mock grave, his assistant turned out to be very ticklish and couldn't stop laughing.[22] A reviewer called the show a "ridiculous farce."[23]

Jansen's growing notoriety became his downfall: local medical schools actually paid him to leave Washington.[24] "With starvation staring him in the face," as his obituary put it, Jansen's life came to a grim end: he took his own life with a pistol in New York.[25] His age could only be estimated, but at the time of his death he was anywhere from 45 to 50 years old. Jansen once said that he "grimly lamented his inability to rob his own grave of his own body, because no one else could do such things as well."[26]

Perhaps because of his medical background, Jansen saw his work as something he did not just for money, but the advance of science. His obituary in the *Washington Post* read:

> He was born to be a grave robber and followed his trade by instinct. He was most happy in the companionship of corpses...He loved his business, ghastly as

> it was, and followed it with the same enthusiasm that spurs other men to nobler deeds in respectable walks of life. He was proud, strange to say, of this work and glorified in doing it in a systematic, scientific way. He did not belong to that class of grave robbers who steal bodies for ransom, but simply sought to supply medical colleges with subjects for dissection. But even in this lower branch of his profession, so to speak, he had many opportunities to show his nerve and daring and to meet singular and exciting adventures.[27]

With the passage of time, who the body snatchers were and how they operated has become clouded by myths, in part because of sensationalized or embellished depictions of body snatchers in newspapers, medical journals, and other sources. But patterns in the historical record tell us who they really were and how they really operated. The responsibility for securing subjects rested with the instructor, and John Collins Warren, professor of anatomy and surgery at Harvard Medical School, wrote about this responsibility, "No occurrences in the course of my life have given me more trouble and anxiety than the procuring of subjects for dissection in the medical lectures."[28] Most body snatchers were known only to the physicians they supplied; anonymity was better for business.

Students were also known to engage in body snatching, like Edward H. Dixon, who wrote about his experience "resurrectionizing" at New York City's Rutgers Medical College in 1831.[29] When a rival medical school bribed Rutgers' regular resurrectionists to cut off their supply, Dixon and two of his classmates went to their "favorite ground," the potter's field:

> Our rendezvous was at the ferry house, at twelve o'clock; one was to go for the wagon, a couple of shovels, a sort of pry to get off the lid, and a few bunches of straw to cover the suspicious outline of a large salt sack, when on our return we had bagged the game.[30]

Students also turned to body snatching to pay their tuition. A Philadelphia resurrectionist told a reporter in 1879, "Many a good man has paid his way through college by this business. I could name plenty of good doctors who were resurrectionists."[31] One was Henri Le Caron, who went by the alias Charles Morton, a medical student at the Detroit Medical College who snatched bodies from Sandwich, Ontario and sold them to the University of Michigan.[32] After he graduated, Morton became a full-time body snatcher. Harvard Medical School even had a secret society of body snatchers known as the "Spunker Club." Warren was a member, as was his father John Warren, who founded the medical school.

Some physicians snatched bodies not just to supply their class, but for their own study. Samuel D. Gross was a prominent 19th-century surgeon, immortalized in Thomas Eakins's famous painting *The Gross Clinic* (on display in the Philadelphia Museum of Art). After he graduated from Jefferson Medical College in 1828, Gross practiced in Philadelphia, but it wasn't long before he moved back to his hometown of Easton, Pennsylvania.[33] When a man died by suicide there in 1833, the night he was buried Gross told a University of Pennsylvania medical student visiting Easton, "Green, I want that fellow," and they made their way to the potter's field.[34] But as they began to dig they realized that the soil was filled with gravel, which made their work dangerously noisy. To avoid detection, they gave up and tried to cover their tracks. Not long after, the brother of the man they tried to resurrect crossed paths with Green and accused him of stealing the body, to which he replied that he was free to believe whatever he pleased.[35] When bodies were hard to come by in Easton, Gross "provided himself with a subject by driving in a buggy all the way from Easton to Philadelphia and back with a gruesome companion."[36]

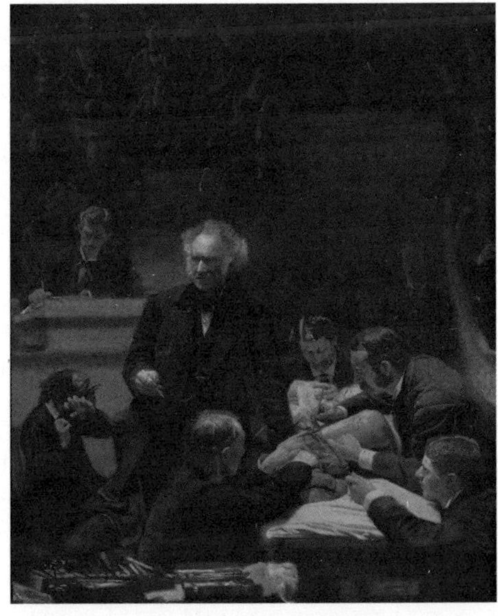

The Gross Clinic, by Thomas Eakins (1875). Samuel D. Gross instructs Jefferson Medical College students. (Wikimedia Commons)

Starting around 1825 physicians began to pay "professional" body snatchers like Cunningham and Jansen to assume the risks of the medical profession's dirty work.[37] There was no clear dividing line between these entrepreneurs and medical men. Anatomists continued to trade the scalpel for the spade if the need and opportunity arose, but they avoided it if they could, as Arthur E. Peticolas wrote to his fellow Virginia physician John Staige Davis in 1856:

> Three weeks before Christmas, our friend [a body snatcher], who had done nothing for some time, disappeared sending a message that he did not care to continue in the business. To continue my lectures I was forced to play resurrectionist myself; by no means a pleasant profession, when the snow is 8 inches deep and the thermometer near zero.[38]

Body snatching was a means to an end for the medical community, a repugnant way to obtain the raw material of science that was fraught with risk: of violence, legal liability, and reputational harm. For professional resurrectionists, body snatching was a lucrative business. While physicians distanced themselves from the trade by hiring middlemen, they were no less responsible for the underground market for bodies they created and fueled.

Professional body snatchers normally had other employment for the off-season, since they only operated when medical schools were in session. According to historian Ruth Richardson, at least in London, most body snatchers didn't start out as criminals but had an occupation associated with the dead: gravedigger, cemetery superintendent, or employment in a medical school or hospital.[39] Some worked in transportation, which was a convenient cover: if your job really was to transport cargo or people, it would be less suspicious if you were seen driving a wagon at night. Body snatching was seen as a lower-class occupation, one that "bummers, outcasts, derelicts only will engage in," according to a 19th-century physician.[40]

Whether by a professional, a physician, or a medical student, body snatching was carried out in similar ways. A successful body snatching required planning, and the first step was to gather information. The best way to find out when and where the dead were buried was from the source: cemetery staff. With someone on the inside, body snatchers had access not only to information but the cemetery itself, where they could carry out their work without fear of detection. Sometimes cemeteries saved body snatchers the trouble of digging up bodies at all. Many coffins that family and friends of the dead believed contained their loved ones were already empty or filled with rocks to give the impression that they rested inside. An undertaker in Grand Rapids, Michigan, held a fake funeral for a destitute man entrusted to him by the county superintendent and sold the body after.[41] He fled the town before his trial. When two New York medical schools competed over bodies in the early 1830s, "Whoever bid highest to induce the keeper of Potter's Field to tie up his dogs, get drunk, and go quietly to bed, was allowed to monopolize the pauper bodies."[42] Bribing cemetery staff cut into profits, and it was worth every penny, but not everyone could be bought. If it wasn't an inside job, body snatchers had to get creative. Body snatchers targeted cemeteries on the periphery of cities or towns, away from prying eyes but still reasonably close to the medical school they planned to visit before dawn.

The local newspaper's death notices, or obituaries section, was one way to find a prospective body.[43] Body snatchers also cultivated networks of informants. A "spy network" was in place at the University of Michigan in the 19th century that informed the demonstrator of anatomy when people died in public institutions who were unclaimed.[44] Former medical students were known to stay in contact with their *alma mater* and sent messages about recent burials.[45]

Body snatchers also needed to know exactly where the body was interred in the cemetery; they might just *happen* to be hunting near a cemetery during a funeral, while they actually noted the burial location.[46] Washington, D.C. body snatcher George Christian called this kind of reconnaissance "prospecting," which he wrote about in his diary, excerpts of which were published in newspapers after his arrest:

> Oct. 29.—Attended a funeral at the Congressional Cemetery this afternoon and brought the subject in to College to-night.
>
> Nov. 9th—Sunday.—Dr. Schlimer went out riding this afternoon, hoping to see a funeral, but were not so fortunate as to meet one.[47]

Physicians only paid for fresh subjects, ideally within a day of burial, and never more than three; a body would be completely decomposed in 10 days.[48] This also depended on the weather, as the heat would putrefy them faster, while the cold would slow the process. There were some tell-tale signs of a newly dug grave. Family and friends left fresh flowers or other mementos. The soil was also loose and unsettled, which made digging easier, and a mound of dirt was sometimes left atop the grave to prevent grave sinking (the process of dirt settling in the grave as air escapes from the soil).[49] In an old grave the dirt was compacted, which made digging especially difficult. Some body snatchers used these signs to find bodies to steal, such as Cunningham; his assistant Charles Keeton told a reporter:

> We go to the "poor lots," the Potter's Field, and when we can find any fresh graves we get the bodies…When we'd come through to the part where the graves were close together, and we knew it was the poor lot where the people without any friends are buried, then we'd dig down to the coffin.[50]

Body snatchers generally targeted public burial grounds, which drew less attention if caught and were generally less well protected. A body snatching from a "respectable" graveyard could become national news, while one from the potter's field may brook resistance but was less likely to become a scandal. Black cemeteries were another common target of body snatchers.

It was difficult to know just by looking at a grave when it was dug, and if the bodies inside would be fresh enough to sell. Christian also learned the hard way that it was difficult to find anything in the dark of night: "Nov. 19.—Went out to the alms house to-day and stayed until evening, expecting to get a subject that was buried to-day. When we went down after dark, however, we found it not, on account of the darkness."[51]

Christian's associate Maude Pratt had a particularly ingenious way of "prospecting." She attended funerals posed as a mourner:

> Heavily veiled and decked out in the most sombre looking dress, weeping as though her heart were broken, Maude would accompany the family to the cemetery; she always wanted a few flowers from the coffin of the dead friend; she would by some unfortunate accident drop these flowers near the grave and then report progress. The position of the flowers usually showed the right grave.[52]

Others pretended to be the family of the deceased, to claim them in public institutions, such as the Edinburgh resurrectionist "Merry Andrew":

> Marvellous were the expedients resorted to by these false claimants of the unprotected dead, and equally marvellous was their success…When assuming

> the character of mourner, his appearance was dismal enough; his pale face, with dropped jaw, set off by the habiliments of grief, and odd manner, far surpassed any theatrical "get up."...After dwelling on the virtues of his "dear relative," he would at length intimate that he wished to convey "the remains" to the family burial-place in the country; that he and some friends would return with a cart and coffin towards evening.[53]

Merry even held a fake funeral procession with his associates, which included a "mock minister" dressed as a clergyman. After they got paid by the anatomist, they had a night on the town and got "dead drunk."[54]

Gathering information was only one of many steps in planning a "night expedition," as Christian called it. While physicians and students supplied themselves, professional body snatchers needed a buyer. It was best to have one already lined up to deliver it to the same night: the faster it was dissected, the faster the evidence of their incursion was destroyed, and the faster it was delivered, the fresher it was. Some physicians had informal arrangements with body snatchers, while others had formal contracts, as an 1849 letter to John Staige Davis indicated: "It would be better if you would state how many subjects you would want at a time, and at what intervals, for though a contract of this sort could not be followed litterally [*sic*], owing to the incidents of the trade, yet something of the kind would be advantageous to steer by."[55]

Body snatching was not a one-person job. A team had to be assembled, ideally with three members: a driver (someone with a wagon), a lookout, and at least one to do the snatching. Larger groups drew more attention, and profits had to be split more ways, which reduced each person's earnings. Conditions had to be right for a body snatching to be successful. The weather had to be agreeable. Rain made the soil difficult to dig, and snow created obvious tracks if it ended before their work was done.[56] If the soil was frozen, digging would be challenging, if not impossible. It was often said that body snatchers avoided plying their trade during a full moon. The London resurrectionist Joseph Naples once wrote in his diary, "the moon at the full, could not go," and the back of one page included notes on "Rules for finding the moon on any given day."[57] In a dense city like London, darkness was the body-snatcher's friend, not the bright light of the moon. It was less of an issue when stealing a body in a remote, unprotected graveyard.

Many body snatchers drank alcohol before, during, and after a snatch. While it became a trope of body-snatching stories, there was some truth to it. Whether they drank to fortify their spirits or to dull their senses for the grim work, or had a drinking problem like Cunningham and Jansen, was unclear. The infamous Edinburgh body-snatcher William Burke "could not sleep without a bottle of whisky by his bed-side… When he wakened, sometimes in fright, he would take a draught at the bottle, often to the extent of half of its contents at a time, and that induced sleep, or, rather, stupor."[58] As one might expect, alcohol often hindered rather than helped the job. Naples, a member of the London Borough Gang of body snatchers, wrote about how it often got in the way of their work:

> *Tuesday 21st.* Look'd out, Jack & Butler drunk as before, hindred [*sic*] us of going out. At Home.
>
> *Wednesday 26th.* Went to look out. Could not go out Jack and Tom got drunk.[59]

Body snatchers required certain tools to complete their task. A shovel was of course needed to dig. Wooden ones were preferred over metal to dampen their noise, especially when digging in rocky soil. An implement was needed to pry coffins open, such as a crowbar (an ax or saw was too noisy), or an auger was used to bore holes in the coffin.[60] Another tool was used to pull the body out by the neck or arms, such as a rope or hook. Finally, a lantern was needed to see, preferably a shaded or "dark lanthorn"—used by burglars and other criminals at the time—which had a sliding shutter to adjust how much light the candle emitted.[61] Sometimes body snatchers even made makeshift tents over the grave to hide the light they generated from passersby.[62]

One of the most common misconceptions of body snatching was that the entire grave needed to be unearthed to reach the coffin. In reality, only a small portion of the earth needed to be removed: the area near the head of the body, which had to be dug deep and wide enough to be able to clamber down and break open the coffin, perhaps two or three feet square. The location of the body's head wasn't hard to locate because they were, and are, commonly positioned in front of the headstone. In Christian cemeteries the headstone also generally

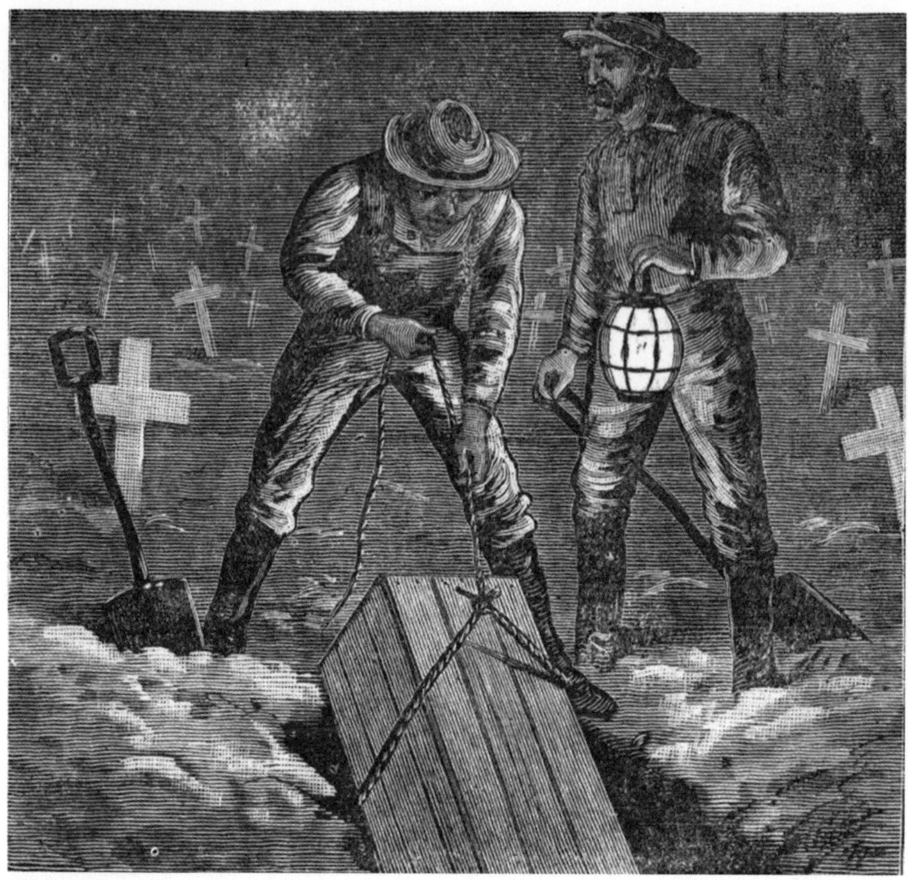

Body snatchers unearth a coffin. Normally, they dug a hole near the head of the grave and used it to break open the coffin to remove the body. (National Library of Medicine)

faces east, the direction from which it is believed Christ will appear in the Second Coming.

Despite the popular phrase "six feet under," there is no standard grave depth. The phrase came from a London mayor in 1665 who ordered that all graves in the city be buried 6 feet deep, which he believed would help stop the spread of the plague. Today coffins in Pennsylvania must be a minimum of 1.5 feet below the ground, which varies from state to state, as it did in the past. But the shallower the grave, the faster it was for a body snatcher to get to the coffin.

Another myth was the idea that body snatchers tunneled into the grave, which was featured in a medical journal in 1896:

> Several feet—fifteen or twenty—away from the head or foot of the grave he would remove a square of turf about eighteen or twenty inches in diameter. This he would carefully put by, and then commence to mine. Most pauper graves were of the same depth, and if the sepulchre was that of a person of importance the depth of the grave could be pretty well estimated by the nature of the soil thrown up. Taking a five-foot grave, the coffin lid would be about four feet from the surface. A rough slanting tunnel some five yards long would, therefore, have to be constructed so as to impinge exactly on the coffin head. This being at last struck (no very simple task), the coffin was lugged up by hooks to the surface, or, preferably, the end of the coffin was wrenched off with hooks while still in the shelter of the tunnel, and the scalp or feet of the corpse secured through the open end and the body pulled out, leaving the coffin almost intact and unmoved. The body once obtained, the narrow shaft was easily filled up and the sod of turf accurately replaced. The friends of the deceased, seeing that the earth *over* his grave was not disturbed, would flatter themselves that the body had escaped the resurrectionist; but they seldom noticed the neatly placed square of turf some feet away.[63]

This implausible method had many problems. For a task in which speed was of the essence, it would have taken too long: a graveyard's compacted soil was harder to dig than a fresh grave's loose soil, and digging a tunnel was of course more time-consuming than digging a hole atop a grave. The location of the head of the grave told body snatchers where the head of the body was, but judging the depth of the grave and the angle of the tunnel was a crapshoot. Even if someone managed to pull it off, dragging the coffin through the tunnel was unrealistic at best. If the reason for this elaborate workaround was to leave no evidence above a grave, a hole in a graveyard not associated with a burial plot might be even more suspicious to cemetery staff. Tunneling was more practical as a method of escaping prison than snatching a body.

During the digging a tarp was sometimes placed next to the grave to toss the dirt on so that when it was returned none would be left behind, an obvious sign that the grave had been disturbed.[64] Above all else, avoiding detection was paramount. If caught, body snatchers faced vigilante justice, jail time, and fines, but if they didn't have someone on the inside they also lost their supply, as the cemetery would then be on high alert.

The lookout might throw tiny pebbles to quietly signal that someone was approaching.[65] John Collins Warren recalled a close call during a body snatching as a student at Harvard Medical School in 1796.[66] His resurrection party reached the wall of the cemetery with a body, but a man on the other side was smoking. He must have been smoking for a long time, because one of the body snatchers did something counterintuitive: he pretended to be intoxicated and picked a fight with the man. Another body snatcher approached and came to the stranger's defense, ending the fake fight, and ensuring that the stranger went on his way past the cemetery and the body snatching in progress. Warren returned to the grave to hide the evidence of their incursion: "I, knowing the importance of covering up the grave and effacing the vestiges of our labor, remained, with no very agreeable sensations, to finish the work."[67] No matter how much planning body snatchers did, there were many things out of their control that could go wrong, which required an ability to improvise.

Digging was taxing work, and the lookout and the watchman might take turns as one became tired. One body snatcher said, "accustomed as he had been to hard labour all his life, he had no idea of any exertion comparable with that which was required in these 'jobs,' as he called them."[68] With the hole dug, the head of the coffin would then be broken open. Since only the head of the grave was dug, the dirt holding down the rest of the coffin provided the necessary leverage to open the casket with a crowbar.[69] Breaking the coffin open could be noisy, as one body snatcher recalled:

> I was one of four who had agreed to exhume the body of a man of immense size. After procuring the necessary pick and spades, rope and sack, we proceeded to the designated place of burial. But the light from the surrounding windows fell brightly on the tomb-stones, and rendered it unsafe, at so early an hour, to engage in the execution of our task. Wrapped in our cloaks, we lay concealed in the dark shadows of the church, until after midnight. Then we assumed the duties assigned to us. One was stationed at the entrance, another at the outlet of the graveyard, as sentinels, while a third and myself commenced the digging. No countersign was given of approaching danger, until we reached the lid of the coffin. It was made of thick boards, and fastened with long screws, so that much force was required to break it. It gave way with a loud noise, which resounded from house to house, and roused the faithful watch-dogs from their slumbers. A general barking ensued, lamps were lighted, and forms were dimly seen, passing

> the windows. Not a footstep, however, was heard approaching us, and we returned to our labour, which had been temporarily suspended.[70]

Body snatchers sometimes covered up the coffin to dampen the noise generated by breaking it open.[71] In the potter's fields that body snatchers targeted most frequently, coffins were generally built using cheap materials that posed little obstacle in forcing them open. In places like Philadelphia's almshouse, mass graves with multiple coffins were stacked on top of each other and only lightly buried, making it easier for body snatchers to take the bodies graveyard attendants sold.

When the coffin was opened, depending on the level of decomposition, the smell would have been pungent. A rope or a hook was then placed around the neck or under the arms of the corpse, and the body was pulled out and placed in a sack (hence the body-snatcher's nickname, the sack-'em-up men). However, the shape of coffins, which were usually narrower at the head and the feet and resembled the shape of the body, presented a challenge when pulling it out with only the head of the coffin exposed (the modern American casket is rectangular, which does not have this problem). As a body snatcher explained it, they overcame this challenge by "rounding the shoulders well over the chest, and then in drawing out the body, giving it such a general turn as to be enabled at once to extract it in the diagonal of the opening already described."[72]

Once out of the grave, according to a Philadelphia body snatcher, the body was doubled up in the sack "nose and knee like."[73] By the time the body was stolen, it may or may not have been affected by rigor mortis—a temporary stiffening of the body's limbs—but placing it in a sack would be much more difficult if it was. Any clothing or valuables were taken off the corpse and placed back into the coffin: they were only there to steal the body, and it was best not to keep anything that could later be used to identify the body. The dirt was returned to the grave, but not before the coffin lid; otherwise the dirt would fill the empty coffin and create a sinkhole (tunneling to the grave and pulling the coffin out underground also risked this).[74]

Getting away with the body was not enough. If done right, no trace was left behind that the grave had been disturbed. Otherwise, people would put two and two together and check the local college, which got them and their body snatchers in hot water. Some claimed that body snatchers could complete the process in as little as 15 minutes, and that they could steal as many as six in one night.[75] On average it took under an hour to take one "stiff," but the length of time depended on many factors, such as the depth of the grave.

The body was then loaded for transport. Carrying the body to the wagon couldn't have been easy. As decomposition sets in, the body of a deceased person weighs less than when they were alive: it only seems as if they weigh more because they are, literally, dead weight. Hand-holds could be attached to the sacks bodies were placed in to make them easier to carry.[76] A wagon outside a cemetery at night was a giveaway that something nefarious was going on, so unless it could be well hidden, the driver might arrive at an appointed time when the body snatching was expected to be done.[77] They might also drive in a loop and wait for the lookout to give a signal to stop. Rufus Cantrell, the "King of Ghouls" who led a group of body snatchers in Indianapolis, had a wagon that "was a three-seated conveyance with a canopy top and side curtains. The tools were inside and it was often true that work on two or three graves

Height Im. 76.9
" 5 Ft.10 in.
Outs A. Im. 93.0
Trunk. 89.9
Head lgth. 20.5
" width. 16.3
Cheek width 14.9
R. Ear. 6.0
L. Foot. 27.5
L. Mid. F. 12.7
L. Lit. F. 9.9
L. Fore A. 51.7
2670

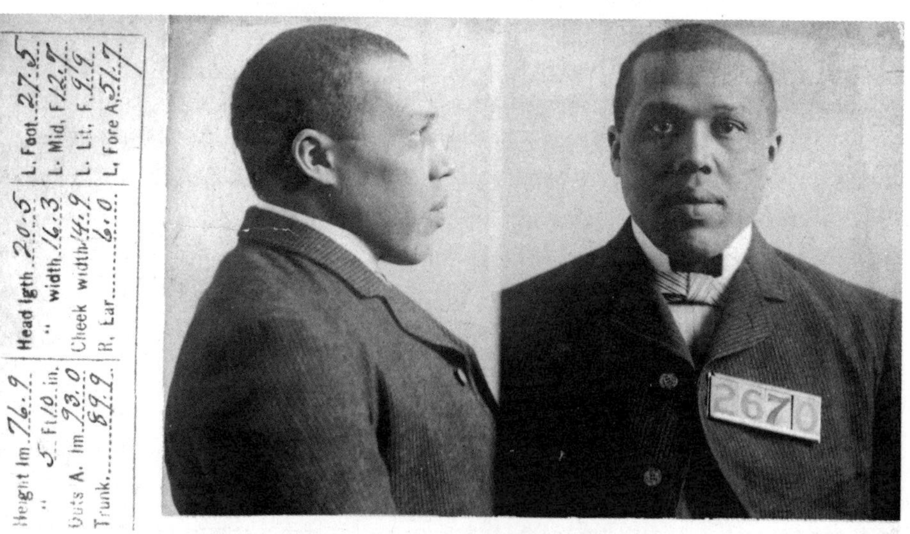

1903 mugshot of Rufus Cantrell, the "King of Ghouls" who operated in Indianapolis, as well as Philadelphia. (Indiana Archives and Records Administration)

was going on at the same time."[78] Cantrell also operated for a time in Philadelphia, and once shipped a body to the city from Indianapolis.[79]

After loading the body and carefully hiding it in the carriage, it was delivered to a medical school. Transporting bodies had its own set of risks. The night watch was one threat, but they could sometimes be bribed, as a story in an American newspaper indicated:

> On one occasion, a student was conveying a subject, carefully packed in a hamper, in a hackney-coach, from one hospital to another. To his surprise and alarm, the coach stopped in front of the police office. The coachman descended from his box, and putting his face in at the window, said in a low but significant tone: "Sir, my fare to the place you want to go to is $10, unless you wish to be put down here." The student took the hint, and paid the money.[80]

Upon delivery, and most importantly, when they were paid, the body-snatcher's work was complete. Body snatching was a profitable business that could fetch a month's worth of wages in one night.[81] But as with any market, prices fluctuated. If bodies were plentiful, such as in times of war, it plummeted. If bodies were scarce, it spiked. The types of bodies also affected the price. For Virginia physician John Staige Davis, a mother and her child (which may have referred to a pregnant woman) commanded the highest price, followed by adults (14 or above), eight- to 10-year-olds, and infants (up to eight years old), while "Dropsical [swollen with fluid] or very obese subjects are not to be furnished."[82] Even today many medical schools turn away whole body donations based on a person's BMI (body mass index) due to the difficulty of moving larger corpses and the additional adipose tissue (body fat) to cut through; by the standards of some colleges, the average American male is too overweight to be accepted for dissection.[83] Pennsylvania's Humanity Gifts Registry, which handles body donations for all medical schools in the state, lists on its website that it doesn't accept "obese" bodies.[84] Some consider such rejections a bias, and that bodies the students practice on in medical schools should be representative of the general population, which would improve care.

Curious medical cases were particularly valuable. In New York, around 1868, a woman whose affliction stumped the physicians who treated her died.[85] The physicians wanted to dissect the woman to try to learn more about her condition, but her family wouldn't allow it. They hired body snatchers to assist them and resurrected the woman. Ultimately, the price of bodies was negotiable, and when they had leverage, body snatchers could drive a hard bargain, as one story in an American newspaper retold:

> At the commencement of a certain session, one Murphy, a noted character, presented himself before the house-surgeon. After some unimportant conversation, he said:
>
> "Well, doctor, this season I must have $100 down, and $46 for every 'thing' I bring you."
>
> ("Thing" was the cant phrase for "body.")
>
> "Nonsense," replied the surgeon; "'tis downright extortion. I shall employ some one else."
>
> "Very well, sir," said Murphy, turning on his heel; "but you won't be able to do without us."
>
> The event proved that Murphy was right. The new men were either bribed off by the old gang, or else were exposed and detected by the police; so the doctors, in despair, were obliged to re-employ Mr. Murphy.[86]

A letter to John Staige Davis also shed light on difficult negotiations with body snatchers: "With all his vulgarity he seems to be a most able diplomatist, and I confess myself outdone by him, at least as far as closing your bargain goes. It seems he is an old trafficker and perfectly understands the business, as well as taking care of his own interest."[87]

Bodies weren't the only way body snatchers made money. "Extremities," or body parts, were also sold, as Christian wrote about in his diary: "April 4th.—Dr. C. and I went to the Washington Asylum Cemetery to-night and confiscated two sets of extremities and one head."[88] Some also sold the teeth of corpses. An issue of the Baltimore *Saturday Visitor* in 1833 described the practice of stealing teeth from corpses in the grave for dentures.[89] Joseph Naples, the London body snatcher, also wrote multiple times about selling "canines," or teeth: "*Tuesday 24th*...Jack sold the Canines to Mr. Thomson for 5 Guineas."[90] In the 18th and 19th centuries there was an active "tooth trade" in which teeth would be sold by the poor to the rich, pulled without anesthetic for money, or taken from corpses.[91] The increasing availability of sugar further contributed to tooth loss, and at the time the best dentures were made out of human teeth. The teeth of the living or the dead were equally useful for dentures.

George Washington had famously bad teeth. Although the myth of him having wooden teeth is not true, by the time he was inaugurated president in 1789 he had only one real tooth in his mouth, the rest a combination of human teeth, cow, horse, ivory, lead, copper, or silver, and some of the human teeth may have come from enslaved African Americans.[92] After the Battle of Waterloo, Napoleon Bonaparte's final defeat on the battlefield, in what is now Belgium in 1815, teeth were taken from the bodies of dead soldiers. Human teeth were used until about the mid-19th century when better alternatives emerged, but until then it was a lucrative sideline for body snatchers; how widespread the practice was is unknown.[93] There is less evidence of the practice, but some say body snatchers sold the hair of corpses. If there was a way to make money off a body, body snatchers would try.

The most infamous case of body snatching in history technically wasn't a case of body snatching at all. William Burke and William Hare were two Irishmen who immigrated to Scotland. Hare ran a lodging house with his wife Margaret Laird, where Burke lived with his common-law wife Helen McDougal. Burke and Hare met in 1827 and quickly became friends. Later that same year a lodger named Donald died suddenly in the house. Upset that he hadn't fully paid his rent, Burke and Hare realized that they could sell the man's body to anatomists to recoup the cost, which they did, to Dr. Robert Knox's private anatomy school in Surgeon's Square. The pay was good and Knox didn't ask questions, but what started as a happy accident became something much darker.

Burke and Hare could have become body snatchers, but the practice had been a scourge of Edinburgh for some time, and graveyard defenses—such as cemetery watches and mortsafes (cages on graves)—made the job difficult. Instead, over the next 10 months, Burke and Hare killed at least 16 people in a murder spree to sell their bodies for medical education. First, the pair plied their victims with alcohol in their lodging house and made merry, waiting until their victim was drunk to make their move. When they were ready, one put their weight on the victim's chest to hold them down, while the other smothered them. Their method of murder left no evidence, and there was no fresher body than one who had just died, or in this case, had just been killed.

Their last victim was Margaret Docherty, an Irishwoman who came to Edinburgh to find her son.[94] Burke ran into her at a grocery store, where she sought help, and he started a conversation with her. She was the ideal victim: "an old and frail stranger" unknown to anyone in Edinburgh.[95] Burke claimed that his mother's last name was also Docherty and convinced her to come back to his lodging house for breakfast, where instead of receiving the kindness of a stranger she fell victim like so many others. Burke and Hare got away with their crimes until a lodger in the house discovered the body of Margaret Docherty and reported it to the police.

Before the authorities arrived, Burke and Hare sold the body to Dr. Knox. There was enough circumstantial evidence for them to be arrested, but no hard proof, which left the police with one option: to

"Hark! the Doctor knocks – she is almost done – and ready for you –
BURKING POOR OLD Mrs CONSTITUTION Aged 141

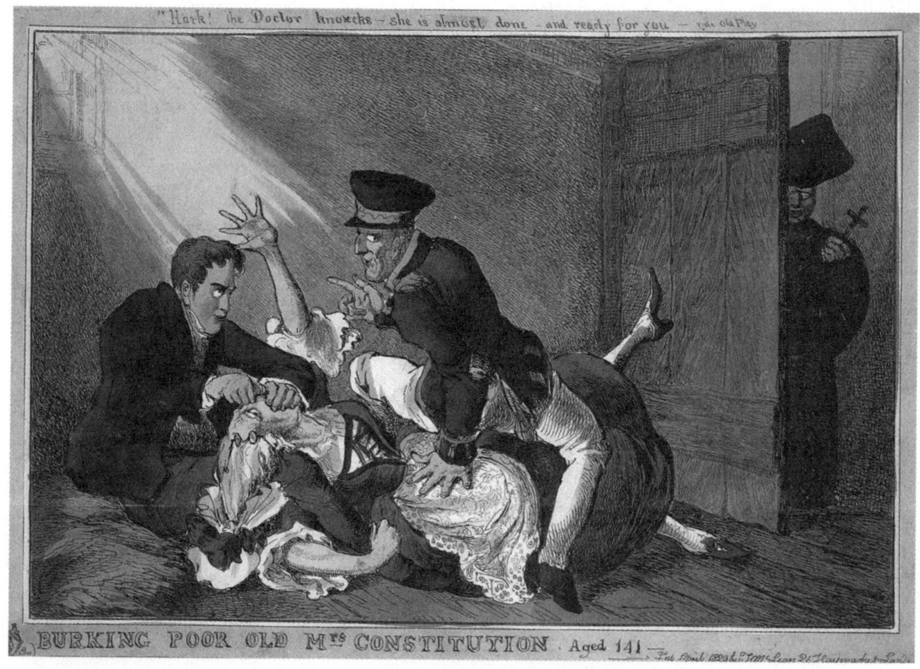

William Burke and William Hare murder Margaret Docherty to sell her body to science, 1829. (Wellcome Collection)

get either Burke or Hare to turn King's evidence—to tell the truth in exchange for immunity from prosecution. Hare did so and went free, while Burke was put on trial and sentenced to death. Burke's partner Helen McDougal was acquitted due to a lack of evidence. After Burke's execution he was, ironically, dissected. His skeleton can be viewed today in the University of Edinburgh's Anatomical Museum, and other objects were made using his skin, including a pocketbook.

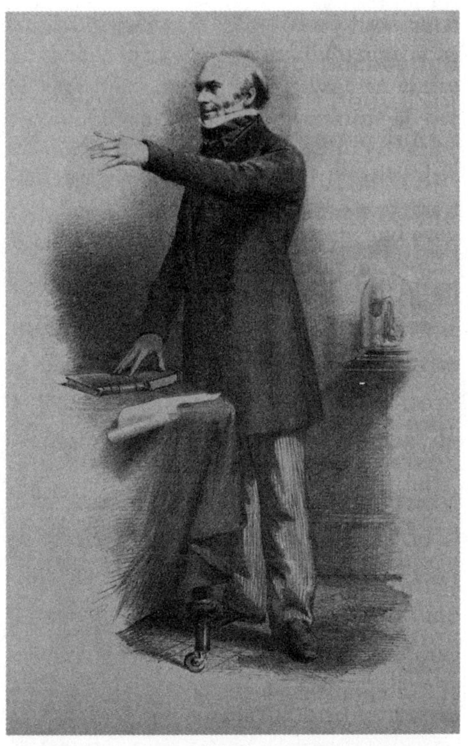

Robert Knox purchased Burke and Hare's ill-gotten bodies for his anatomy classes. (Wellcome Collection)

While Dr. Knox didn't face legal liability, he faced judgment in the court of public opinion: an effigy of Knox was burned in front of his home. "Burke's the butcher, Hare's the thief, Knox the boy that buys the beef," as the rhyme went. His reputation in tatters, Knox moved to London after the death of his wife where he spent the rest of his days. The fate of Hare is unknown. Burke and Hare never stole a body from a grave, and a new word was invented for their crime: "burking," which referred to both murdering for dissection, and their unique method—suffocation.

Even before Burke and Hare, the idea that people might be murdered for dissection was thought possible, but as the butt of a joke, as in one humorous 1810 story in the *Philadelphia Repertory*:

> A man siting [*sic*] one evening at an alehouse, thinking how to get provision for the next day, saw another, dead drunk, on an opposite bench. A thought instantly struck him; so, going to the landlord, he said "Do not you wish to get rid of this sot?" "Aye, to be sure," returned he; "and half a crown shall speak my thanks." "Agreed," said the other, "get me a sack." A sack was brought, and put

> over the drunken guest. Away trudged the man with his burden, till he came to the house of a noted resurrectionist; when he knocked at the door. "Who's there?" said a voice. "I have brought you a subject," replied the man, "so come, quick, give me my fee." The money was immediately paid, and the sack, with its contents, deposited in the surgery. The motion of quick walking had nearly recovered the poor victim, who, before the other had been gone five minutes, began to extricate himself from the sack. The purchaser, enraged at being thus outwitted, ran after the man who had deceived him, collared him, and cried, "Why you dog, the man's alive!" "Alive!" answered the other, "so much the better, kill him when you want him."[96]

Burking was rare, but it was not unheard of after Burke and Hare, outside of Edinburgh. In 1884 the house of the Taylor family burned down in Cincinnati, Ohio, where Beverly Taylor, his wife Elizabeth, and their granddaughter Emma J. Lambert lived.[97] No bodies were found in the wreckage. The family wasn't suspected as the source of the fire, and the marshal ruled out murder or robbery, but he wondered if body snatching might have been the motivation.[98] Sure enough, three bodies were delivered to a local medical school the same night as the fire, and by their appearance seemed to have been beaten to death. The perpetrators were body snatchers—and now murderers—Allen Ingalls and Ben Johnson, who did it for the money the crime would bring. They came in the night, brutally murdered the family, and transported their bodies to the local medical school like the others they previously snatched from graves. Ingalls took his own life before his execution in his cell, while Johnson was hanged.[99] Beverly, one of the victims, had previously been a body snatcher and was rumored to have worked for Cunningham.[100]

In Baltimore in 1886 a woman named Emily Brown was murdered by John Thomas Ross, who worked "in the brick-yards and driving carts" and was the 28-year-old son of Mary Blockson, the owner of the lodging house she was staying in.[101] Brown came from a prosperous family but descended into poverty and addiction; she often failed to pay her rent and resorted to panhandling.[102] Anderson Perry also lived in the house, a janitor at the University of Maryland's School of Medicine, and Blockson's partner. One night Ross murdered Brown with a blow to the head, stabbed her for good measure, and sold her body to the medical school Perry worked at. The physicians who examined her body noticed that not only was it still warm, but it had blood on it and signs of violence. They notified the police.

Ross, Perry, and a man named Albert Hawkins who was believed to have assisted in the crime were arrested. Ross confessed and maintained that Perry was the mastermind of the crime, who wanted the 15 dollars they could sell Brown for (a sizable sum at the time), and that Hawkins helped him do it. But with only circumstantial evidence, it was Ross's word against Perry's and Hawkins's, and only he was convicted and executed for the murder of Brown. In his last written statement, Ross lamented:

> I've no excuse to offer,
> My guilt I freely own,
> But does it look like justice
> I must suffer all alone?
> Is it fair, kind Christians,
> In this land of liberty
> That I alone must suffer,
> And the other two go free?[103]

Despite not being body snatchers in the usual sense, the most well-known fictional stories about the practice were inspired by Burke and Hare. In Robert Louis Stevenson's *The Body Snatcher*, a short story published in 1884, the character Fettes studied medicine under a Dr. K (a not-so-subtle reference to Dr. Knox), and was responsible for dealing with body snatchers. Bodies were in short supply, and Dr. K's motto was "They bring the body, and we pay the price," no questions asked.[104] But one night Fettes couldn't help but notice that the body delivered was someone he knew was alive and well the day before; there was no doubt that she had been murdered. Wolfe Macfarlane, the class assistant, told Fettes that all the bodies they received had been murdered, and urged him to stay silent. Despite his guilty conscience, Fettes did what he was told. Later, Fettes and Macfarlane had dinner with a body snatcher named Gray, a "coarse, vulgar, and stupid" man who treated Macfarlane poorly, and had some kind of leverage over him, probably incriminating information about their past dealings.[105]

Not long after, Macfarlane delivered the next body: Gray, whom Macfarlane had murdered. Fettes again reluctantly kept quiet, but as time passed he overcame his inner turmoil: "Hell, God, Devil, right, wrong, sin, crime, and all the old gallery of curiosities—they may frighten boys, but men of the world, like you and me, despise them."[106] After some time Fettes and Macfarlane became body snatchers themselves to steal the body of a woman: "Late one afternoon the pair set forth, well wrapped in cloaks and furnished with a formidable bottle [of alcohol]...They were both experienced in such affairs, and powerful with the spade; and they had scarce been twenty minutes at their task before they were rewarded by a dull rattle on the coffin lid."[107]

They rode into the night with the woman's body propped up between them in a sack, but something was off. When they examined her again in the light they were shocked to discover that the body was Gray's, whom they had already dissected, a real or imagined manifestation of Fettes's and Macfarlane's guilt for their actions.

The story received a Hollywood treatment in the 1945 film of the same name, which starred Boris Karloff—who famously portrayed Frankenstein—as the body snatcher, and featured Bela Lugosi as the medical school's janitor, who famously portrayed Dracula. The film was more focused on Gray, who was a cabman (an older term for taxi driver) by day and a body snatcher at night, without a moral bone in his body, motivated only by money. The plot was similar to Stevenson's short story, but another element was added to raise the stakes: the physicians needed a body to practice on to treat a young girl who needed a risky operation. It was the same moral dilemma anatomists faced:

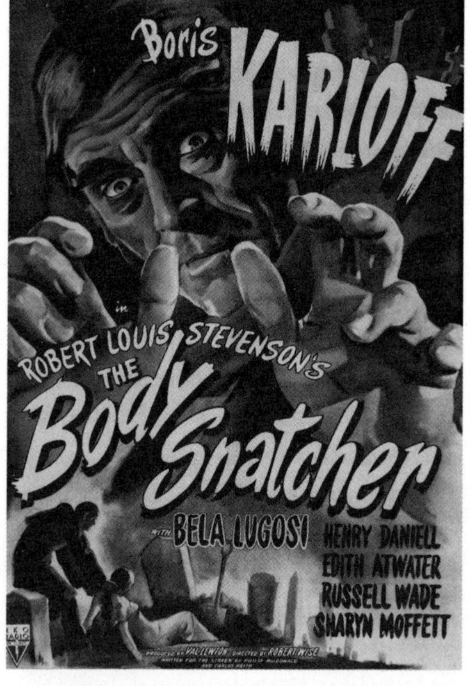

Boris Karloff starred in Hollywood's adaptation of Robert Louis Stevenson's *The Body Snatcher*, 1945. (Wikimedia Commons)

to violate the sanctity of the grave for the progress of science, except in stories like this, body snatchers were also willing to murder for it.

While stories like *The Body Snatcher* may have given the impression that all body snatchers were burkers, few stooped to murder to supply subjects in real life. But the public perception of body snatchers was shaped largely by how they were depicted in popular culture. Other famous stories that featured body snatching were inspired by, or set in, Philadelphia—the center of medicine and body snatching in 19th-century America.

Edgar Allen Poe—one of America's most celebrated writers for his poetry and short stories—moved to Philadelphia in 1838. The melancholic and troubled author spent six years in the city, which were said to be his most prolific and happiest.[108] Until the mid-19th century, Philadelphia was the center of the American book-printing and publishing industry, and Poe came to the city to start a literary magazine.[109]

In 1839 he published *The Fall of The House of Usher*, a story in which an unnamed narrator visits the mansion of his ailing, long-lost childhood friend Roderick Usher. When he arrives, he learns that Roderick's sister Madeline is also sick. Roderick and Madeline are the only remaining members of the Usher family, and Roderick believes that the mansion possesses a kind of sentience and control over them, and that their maladies are related to it. Not long after, Madeline dies. Worried that the family physician is planning to disinter and dissect her, Roderick explains how he intends to preserve the body:

> [He will place] her corpse for a fortnight (previously to its final interment), in one of the numerous vaults within the main walls of the building...by consideration of the unusual character of the malady of the deceased, of certain obtrusive and eager inquiries on the part of her medical men, and of the remote and exposed situation of the burial-ground of the family.[110]

But Madeline isn't actually dead; she escapes her premature burial, after which she attacks Roderick, which scares him to death—literally—and then she also dies. The narrator flees the house as it collapses, which represents the end of the Usher family line. While Poe didn't address body snatching in Philadelphia directly, many of his stories reflect a preoccupation with death, dead bodies, and the medical profession that was emerging in the city he lived in.

However, Poe's friend George Lippard directly addressed body snatching in Philadelphia in his novel *The Quaker City, or The Monks of Monk Hall*, published in 1845. For a time, it was the bestselling novel in America, until the publication of Harriet Beecher Stowe's *Uncle Tom's Cabin* in 1852.[111] The story revolves around Monk Hall, a fictional Philadelphia mansion and the site of a secret club where the city's most powerful citizens meet to engage in all kinds of debauchery: drinking, drugs, seduction, rape, and murder. The book's title was ironic: Philadelphia's Quakers were known for their high moral standards, but the book is actually about hypocritical members of the upper class—seen as upstanding citizens outside of Monk Hall—and the city's dark underbelly.[112] The novel's connection to body snatching is through Monk Hall's doorkeeper, a man known as "Devil-Bug," whose "Soul was like his body, a mass of hideous and distorted energy...To him, there was no such thing as *good* in the world."[113] He is also a body snatcher:

> "The *doctor* sent for me last night; the one what wants me to steal dead bodies for him. I must go airily in the mornin'; he pays me well; and I likes the business. Sich a jolly business! To creep over the wall o' some grave yard in the dead o' the night, and with a spade in yer hand, to turn up the airth of a new made grave! To mash the coffin lid into small pieces with a blow o' the spade, and to drag the stiff corpse out from its restin' place, with the shroud so white and clean, spotted by the damp clay! To kiver the corpse with an old over-coat or a coffee bag, and bear it off to the doctor, with his penknife's and his daggers and his gim'lets! Hoo, hoo!" he emitted a wild imitation of the screech-owl, from his compressed teeth, "sich a jolly business!"[114]

The novel was surprisingly accurate about where bodies for dissection came from in Philadelphia around the time the book was published:

> "From whence did you bring this subject?" said Ravoni in a low whisper.
> "From the poor man's grave in the Alms-house grave-yard," answered the tallest of the Resurrectionists. "Yer honor knows there's one grave which is the property o' the Doctors? Any body what dies in the Almshouse and hai'nt got no friends to claim him, is put into this grave, and the d—l himself may take him if he likes."[115]

That body snatching in Philadelphia was featured in what was once America's most popular novel demonstrates just how widely the city's practice filtered into popular culture. While Poe was paid only a "sawbuck"—10 dollars—for *The Fall of The House of Usher*, and struggled to make ends meet, Lippard was one of the best paid authors of his time.[116] But while Poe is now in the pantheon of America's great authors, Lippard's work has largely been forgotten.

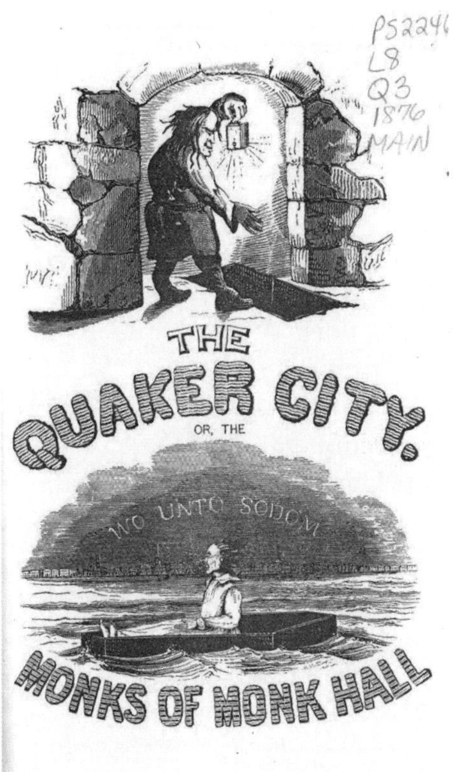

The Quaker City, or The Monks of Monk Hall (1845) was once America's bestselling book, and featured body snatching in Philadelphia. (The Internet Archive)

Body snatchers weren't the amoral fiends or monsters they were depicted as in literature, or "murderers, criminals, desperate fellows" as a 19th-century physician called them.[117] They were people, and to them body snatching was a business transaction like any other. But sometimes the history of body snatching could be stranger than fiction. As the 19th century progressed and body snatching became more widespread—and the number of professional body snatchers grew—the public and the people whose job it was to care for the dead, such as cemetery superintendents, became aware of what the body snatchers were up to and instituted defenses to prevent midnight incursions of the grave. While some were more passive, like cemetery watches or burial vaults, others actively tried to stop body snatchers in their tracks. Later in the century, defenses became more lethal, such as the coffin torpedo, part of an industry developed to defend the dead. Even proponents of cremation, which was not widely practiced in 19th-century America, cited body snatching as one reason not to be interred in cemeteries. It was a time when the living needed protection from the dead.

CHAPTER 5

Defending the Dead

Cemetery Guns, Coffin Torpedoes, and Cremation

> Sleep well sweet angel, let no fears of ghouls disturb thy rest, for above thy shrouded form lies a torpedo, ready to make minced meat of anyone who attempts to convey you to the pickling vat.
>
> —ADVERTISEMENT FOR THOMAS N. HOWELL'S COFFIN TORPEDO[1]

Before it closed in the mid-2010s, the Museum of Mourning Art's collection of *memento mori* in Drexel Hill, Pennsylvania had a unique centerpiece: a cemetery gun. Made by Jurgensen Machine Co. in New York in the 18th or early 19th century, it was a booby trap with a surprisingly sophisticated design.[2] The gun was mounted on a base at the foot of the grave, which faced the head of the grave, connected to three trip wires that—if triggered by an unsuspecting resurrectionist—swiveled it in their direction and fired. Depending on the type of ammunition that was loaded, it could scare off, injure, or even kill intruders.

But to a practiced body snatcher, the grave gun was a mere annoyance: during the day resurrectionists were known to send a "female member of their fraternity" to perform reconnaissance, so that at night they would have "easily found the pegs, and feeling their way cautiously along the wires, they removed the loaded weapon, and pursued their avocation in security."[3] That is, unless cemetery staff caught wind of the scheme and set the trap at night.[4] When the Museum of Mourning Art closed its doors, part of its collection went up for sale on Sotheby's auction house, including the gun. Its condition was listed as fine, with some outdoor use.[5] One can't help but wonder where or when it may have been deployed, if it scared a body snatcher away, or if it was the last thing they ever saw, or heard, before they met their maker.

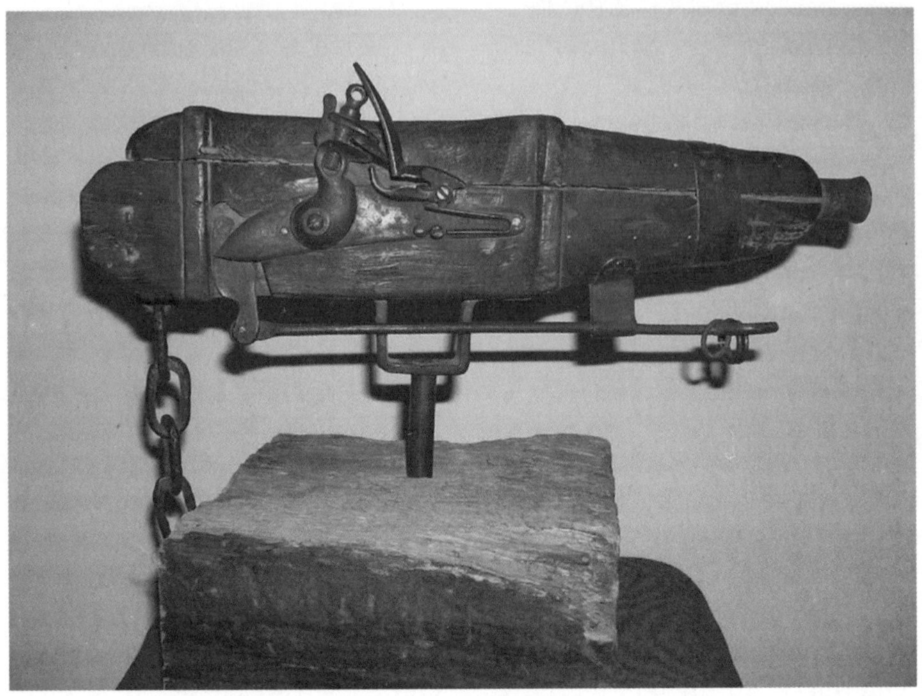

Grave gun from the (now closed) Museum of Mourning Art, a trap placed in cemeteries. (Arlington Cemetery Company)

As medical schools proliferated in 19th-century Philadelphia, so did body snatching, and methods to prevent it. Not all involved deadly weapons, but the fact that devices like the cemetery gun were deployed at all showed how seriously people took the defense of the dead. Some believed the most appropriate punishment for disinterring the dead was death. But as cemeteries employed novel defenses, resurrectionists found equally novel ways around them. After a high-profile body snatching in 1878 became a national scandal, entrepreneurs capitalized on the widespread fear of becoming a subject for the scalpel by making and marketing even more extreme methods of thwarting ghouls—an arms race centered on cemeteries.[6] Around the same time, a then-radical movement challenged the belief in the necessity of burial at all, and proposed a very different solution to preventing body snatching: cremation. A graduate of Philadelphia's Jefferson Medical College, Francis Julius

LeMoyne, established the first crematory in the country in Washington, Pennsylvania, now a historic landmark. Body snatching turned cemeteries into battlegrounds, where the living fought over the dead.

★ ★ ★

In Northeastern Pennsylvania, just south of Catawissa, a black sign with white letters that reads "Hooded Grave Cemetery" marks the site of an unusual burial ground. Its name comes from mysterious structures that cover two of the cemetery's graves: iron cages. Their purpose has been the subject of speculation for years, and was even the basis of the 2013 novel *The Caged Graves* by Dianne K. Salerni. Theories range from the ordinary to the supernatural. With their ornate, birdcage-like appearance, some are convinced they were purely decorative.[7] Others believe they were used to keep animals from digging up bodies, or to keep someone—or something—inside the graves: vampires, werewolves, or witches.[8]

According to local historian Ann F. Diseroad, the cages are actually mortsafes, which were most closely associated with the United Kingdom, especially Scotland, where they were deployed in the early 19th century, and many of them can still be seen today.[9] Because they were expensive and only needed for a limited time, there were mortsafe societies in Scotland that, for a fee, made them available for rent.[10] If Diseroad is right, the hooded graves are the only known surviving mortsafes in the United States. But the cages in Catawissa have a key difference with their possible counterparts in Europe. The *Proceedings of the Society of Antiquaries of Scotland* tells us that mortsafes were "intentionally made very heavy to prevent their removal or destruction by unauthorised persons who might wish to gain access to the bodies they protected."[11]

They were so cumbersome that a tackle—a system of pulleys—was sometimes used to put mortsafes on graves and to remove them once bodies had decomposed enough to render them useless for dissection.[12] What made them difficult to install and remove also made them difficult or impossible for body snatchers to break into. However, Pennsylvania's hooded graves seem nowhere near as weighty as other known mortsafes, and may not have presented as much of an obstacle to determined

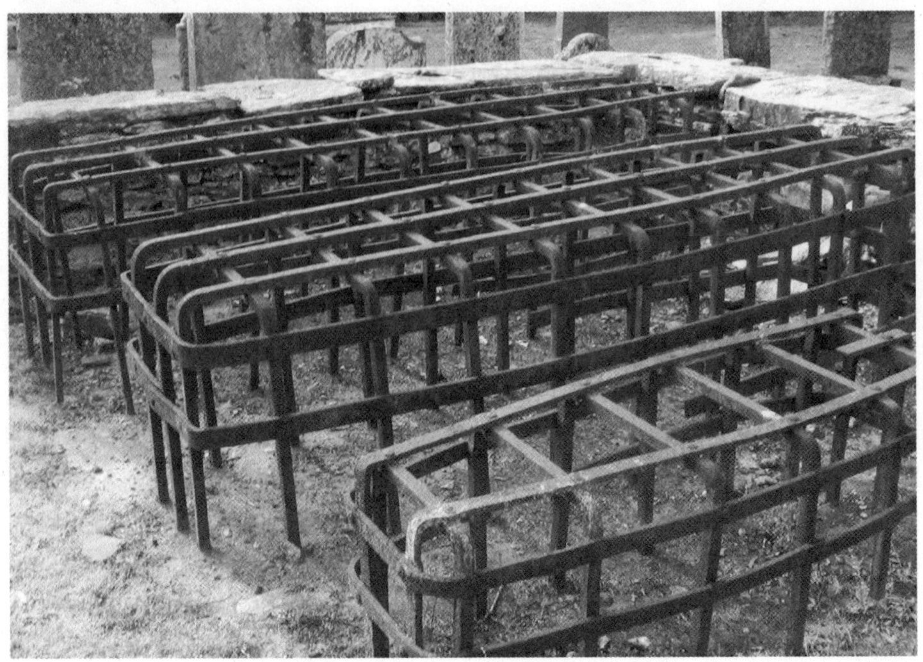

Mortsafes, iron cages placed over graves to prevent disinterment, in Logierait Churchyard, Scotland, in 2006. (Wikimedia Commons / CC BY-SA 3.0)

body snatchers. Despite their differences, there was one feature the hooded graves shared with some mortsafes that point to their true function: padlocks. While they were lost during a restoration, the cages originally had a locking mechanism; why have one if you weren't trying to keep people out?[13]

The occupants of the graves added further to the mystery: two sisters-in-law, Sarah Ann Boone and Asenath Thomas, both died in 1852, possibly of complications from childbirth. A third caged grave was removed in the 1930s by the WPA (the Works Progress Administration, a federal jobs program during the Great Depression) due to disrepair, which may have covered Rebecca Clayton's grave, Sarah's cousin, who died only weeks before the other women, also of an unknown cause.[14] A common factor among the women was that they were part of the Thomas family, which had ties to the iron industry, which may explain the source of the material the cages were made with. But why potentially three women died around the same time, were all related, and had caged graves remains a mystery, unless one of the physicians active in the area planned to snatch their bodies.[15] It's a mystery that will likely remain unsolved, which is why the hooded graves will continue to be a source of fascination.

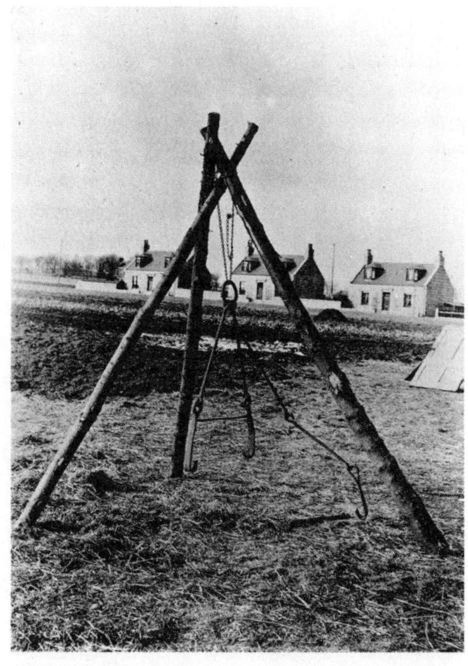
Mortsafe tackle, a system of pulleys used to install and remove mortsafes, at Invererie, Aberdeenshire, in Scotland. (Wellcome Collection / Attribution 4.0 International CC BY 4.0)

Catawissa's caged graves may or may not have been mortsafes, but far simpler means of defending the dead were common in Pennsylvania and across America. Family and friends of course left flowers on graves, but cemetery staff might place other objects like stones in a particular arrangement that, if altered overnight, signaled that the grave had been disturbed.[16] But there was no way to be sure that the grave remained intact if body snatchers "perfectly restored [the objects] to their former position, as to deceive the most anxious visitor to the grave, and, at the first glance, to assure him that all had remained quiet and undisturbed."[17] It was not a foolproof method, but it could fool a less experienced resurrectionist.

Another type of defense was to make disinterment more difficult, which slowed but didn't stop body snatchers; the more time they spent opening a grave, the higher their chance of getting caught. Heavy objects were placed on top of graves, such as large slabs of stone that could only be moved with great effort.[18] Graves could also be dug deeper, and the dirt periodically patted down with a spade while it was filled to create layers of firm soil that made it harder to dig.[19] Others placed objects inside the grave before it was filled, such as planks of wood that could be placed in such a way that made it so the entire grave had to be unearthed.[20]

Freedom's Journal, the first Black-owned American newspaper, wrote in its third issue in 1827:

> As soon as the corpse is deposited in the grave, let a truss of long wheaten straw be opened and distributed in layers, as equally as may be with every layer of earth, until the whole is filled up. By this method the corpse will be effectually secured; as it is certain the longest night will not afford time sufficient to empty the grave, though all the common implements of digging be used for that purpose.[21]

Defenses extended not just to graves, but to the walls and gates that enclosed the graveyards. When Woodlands Cemetery in West Philadelphia was being developed in the first half of the 19th century, there were discussions about how the cemetery should be fortified—by fences or even thorn hedges—given its location near a hotspot of body-snatching activity: Old Blockley, Philadelphia's almshouse.[22] The location of cemeteries mattered, and not just how close they were to medical schools. Starting in the 1830s Philadelphia cemeteries were established farther from the city in more rural areas. Laurel Hill Cemetery (also known as Laurel Hill East) was the second "rural" cemetery established in America, on the banks of the Schuylkill River, as part of what became known as the rural cemetery movement, which featured spacious, park-like cemeteries with ornate monuments. But while rural cemeteries usually had protections like gates, walls, and watchmen, it was actually easier to snatch bodies from them because there were less eyes and ears nearby.[23] The more remote a cemetery was, the more protections it required. And if cemeteries struck secret deals with body snatchers, it was far easier for them to take bodies from remote cemeteries than within dense cities.

Like Philadelphia's almshouse, rural cemeteries erected receiving vaults or dead-houses to store bodies, except they were much more secure. In Philadelphia's West Laurel Hill Cemetery:

> The doors of the receiving-vaults are hermetically sealed. The interior is divided into closets, the doors of which are securely locked, his relatives having one key and the Superintendent the other. The Board of Management have under consideration the idea of running an electric wire between the receiving-vault and the residence of the Superintendent, by which a gong would be sounded in the latter place in the event of any attempt being made to open the vault door.[24]

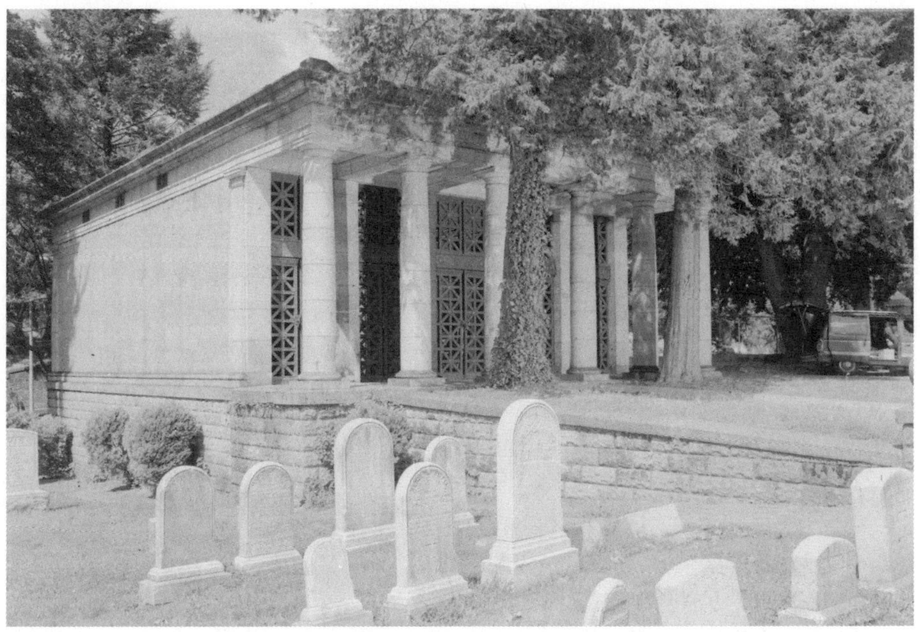

Laurel Hill Cemetery's receiving tomb. (Library of Congress)

George Christian, the D.C. body snatcher, wrote about how he was once stymied by a vault: "Nov. 3d.—Dr. [illegible] and I drove out to Harmony Cemetery this afternoon. Saw some subjects in the vault and went after them tonight but could not get into the place as it was locked."[25] Such structures had multiple functions, such as to temporarily store bodies before funerals or when the ground was too frozen to dig. Bodies were also kept in vaults until they decomposed so that when they were finally buried, the bodies were unsellable, and body snatchers would leave them in peace. Receiving vaults were most commonly used in Philadelphia cemeteries when someone died of an unusual ailment. If families didn't allow physicians to perform an autopsy, they feared—rightly—that physicians might take them from the grave.[26]

Stories abound of physicians going to great lengths to obtain such bodies. A man once died of a curious disease in Washington Asylum, an almshouse in Washington, D.C., which had a "secure place, with windows barred, door locked and chained, almost impossible of burglarious entrance," to store the body.[27] Still, the superintendent didn't believe the body would be safe in the dead-house, and instead put it in his own office. That same night, two medical students came to visit, and more followed. The superintendent thought the students just wanted his company, but when he went to get food for his guests, "the body was lowered from the window into the arms of waiting students and carried away."[28]

One of the most common defenses was the watchman. Some were employed by Laurel Hill Cemetery: "the grounds are patrolled all night by an armed watchman, who is required to be at certain points at certain hours, and to report on a registering apparatus placed in four sections of the grounds at specified intervals."[29] Families and friends also hired watchmen, such as the watch placed over the body of a wealthy man named Thomas Powers in Woodlands Cemetery: "From morning till night a tall, muscular-proportioned man, clad in ulster, can be seen standing near the railing which incloses the lot wherein the remains of the deceased millionaire and his son, who died in 1873, are interred."[30] The mere presence of watchmen acted as a deterrent, but given that only a small window of time was needed for body snatching to happen—less than an hour—they still had to be on high alert. Recent graves were of course the focus of protection, as they were the only ones body snatchers were interested in. Dogs were also let loose on the grounds of Philadelphia cemeteries to alert watchmen of intruders.[31]

It took a certain kind of person to be a watchman: "The watchers needed to be brave men, for it was an eerie occupation watching in the stillness of the night among the dead, and doubtless their nerves were often highly strung."[32] An 1883 Philadelphia newspaper claimed that "tombstone madness" was an occupational hazard of watchmen, who risked "lapsing into a state of melancholia perfectly distinct from any other form of insanity."[33] Ideally they were trustworthy and not susceptible to bribes offered by body snatchers to look the other way during their shift, which was what led some family or friends of the deceased to watch the grave themselves, even if the cemetery already employed a watchman.[34] As a young man Dr. Frederick C. Waite was hired as a watchman to protect the grave of a well-known man in Hudson, Ohio, in 1886. Armed with a shotgun, he stood guard for 10 nights—the time it took for a body to fully decompose—and was well paid for the task.[35]

The arms watchmen carried were not just for show. There are many accounts of body snatchers being shot at or killed by watchmen: in 1897 a man was shot dead and his accomplices wounded in Tennessee by "cemetery guardians."[36] There were also false alarms: "a pig which had by some means got into a churchyard [in Scotland] lost its life through its inability to answer the challenge of the alarmed watchers, who therefore fired in the direction whence the sound proceeded."[37] In Salem County, New Jersey in 1884, a man passing by a cemetery was shot, as was the horse he was riding, because nervous grave guards mistakenly took the farmer for a body snatcher.[38]

John Collins Warren, professor of anatomy and surgery at Harvard Medical School, recalled a time when two students whom he charged with getting a body in Boston's almshouse graveyard escaped the watchmen. They observed the watchmen's movements, and just after midnight, when they thought the moment was right, they disinterred a body. But they had been noticed, and the group of watchmen tried to seize the students. One of the students managed to flee on their wagon. The other was caught but managed to escape the guards as he was escorted to the watchhouse, and a second time after he was recaptured. Despite being in good health before the incident, Warren claimed that the student died not long after due to the strain of the escapes, of "hemorrhage from the lungs."[39]

One of the most high-profile cases of body snatching in American history—what became known as the "Harrison Horror"—demonstrated that no number of defenses could stop a determined body snatcher, and led to even more extreme methods of preventing body snatching. An Ohio congressman and farmer, John Scott Harrison was the son of ninth president William Henry Harrison, who had the shortest presidency in U.S. history: he died of pneumonia after just 32 days in office. John passed away in his home suddenly of a stroke on Saturday, May 25, 1878, and was buried the following Wednesday in Congress Green Cemetery in North Bend, Ohio. Extra precautions were taken to protect John's grave because the grave of his nephew, Samuel Augustus Devin, who passed away shortly before him of tuberculosis, had recently been tampered with in the same cemetery.

John's grave was buried deeper than usual and had a "brick vault, with thick walls and a stone bottom," for the casket to be lowered into.[40] As additional protection, three stones covered the casket, the heaviest placed on the head of the grave, and two smaller stones placed at the foot of the grave, all of which was cemented together, and then of course covered with dirt.[41] If that somehow wasn't enough, a watchman named Thomas Linn was also paid 30 dollars to guard the grave for 30 nights.[42] If you could afford it, multiple defenses could be put in place, but even when seemingly nothing was left to chance, it might not be enough.

After John's funeral, Devin's grave was opened to confirm suspicions that it had been disturbed, where they determined, "An auger had been used, probably to avoid making a noise, and the portion of the lid of the coffin over the head and breast loosened by cutting it from the remainder of the lid by boring across a row of auger holes."[43] John Harrison and George Eaton—John's son and grandson—went to the Ohio Medical College in search of Devin's body, accompanied by a detective and two constables with a warrant, based on a report that the college received a suspicious delivery in the middle of the night from a wagon.[44]

Initially the search was unsuccessful, but when Marshall, the college's janitor, went to inform the faculty of the search, he instead went to a room upstairs—presumably to hide evidence—before he noticed he was being followed.[45] It was there that the group noticed a windlass with a rope that descended into the floor through a trap door, strained by something heavy. Detective Snelbaker rotated the windlass' crank to lift the rope and a body emerged from the shaft, hung by the neck. Bodies were delivered to the college through a chute accessible from the outside. It extended from the fifth floor of the building to the cellar, where body snatchers dumped the body, and where they were hoisted up to the dissecting room.

The face of the naked body before them was covered by fabric, but John saw little point in removing it because it was clearly not Devin: it was far too large. But Snelbaker persisted, and when John took the covering off he likely had the biggest shock of his life: before him was not

Devin, but the body of his father, John Scott Harrison, his face "bruised and discolored" with a "ghastly gash in the neck" where embalming fluid had been injected, his beard "cut squarely off beneath the chin."[46]

Back at Congress Green Cemetery it was discovered that resurrectionists had opened John's grave where its defense was weakest: at the foot of the grave, where the smaller stones were placed. The same technique that had been used to open Devin's grave was used on John's: after lifting the stones, holes were bored into the coffin with an auger, and John's body taken out feet-first.[47] The body snatchers must have had inside information, because they would normally have tried to dig at the head of the grave, which would have proven insurmountable given the extremely heavy rock placed there.[48] The watchman appeared to not have been an accomplice, but didn't stand constant vigil over the grave. Linn checked it throughout the night, but the time in between his visits had been enough for the body to be removed. It probably didn't help that Linn didn't believe someone would be bold enough to attempt to break into John's grave so soon after Devin's.[49]

The incident became national news, and the public was horrified by the situation, which drew a spotlight on a practice that didn't receive as much attention when the victim was a less prominent individual. The college's faculty denied any responsibility or knowledge of the affair, but when Marshall, the college's janitor, was arrested for receiving and concealing Harrison's body, the college's faculty posted his bail for a substantial amount of money.[50] Marshall admitted that he worked with the body-snatcher Charles Morton, who used the college's facilities to prepare bodies to ship them elsewhere. Morton was also indicted, but he evaded arrest and was never found. Devin had been shipped to a medical school in Ann Arbor, Michigan, where he was later found, and a volunteer guard of citizens kept watch after he was buried a second time in Congress Green Cemetery, where John was also later re-interred.[51] Benjamin Harrison, one of John's sons, sued the college in civil court for damages, but its outcome, and Marshall's trial, have been lost to history.[52] Benjamin would go on to become the 23rd president of the United States; his deceased father John became the only person in American history to be both the son and father of U.S. presidents.

The case raised many questions without answers. Why was John's body stolen in the first place? Why would Morton or any body snatcher take the risk of stealing such a well-known person, instead of a corpse from the potter's field? Some suggested it was because the nature of John's death piqued the interest of local doctors. Whatever the reason, the message of the "Harrison Horror" at the time was simple: if it could happen to a congressman, it could happen to anyone. Even after instituting all manner of protections, it wasn't always enough. This created an opportunity for entrepreneurs to profit from the widespread fear of body snatching that resulted from the case, which led directly to the invention of even deadlier devices to prevent body snatching.

★ ★ ★

In 1881 a body snatcher served as a lookout while his two companions unearthed a grave in Mount Vernon, Ohio. As the pick of one of the body snatchers hit the earth, it struck something, but it wasn't the coffin. Then the unthinkable happened: an explosion. The body snatcher, named Dipper, was instantly killed, and the other's leg was maimed. The lookout ran to help his surviving accomplice. Together they fled the scene on their wagon, leaving Dipper's body behind, and the dead body they were trying to snatch. The next day's local paper summarized the event with the headline "A Torpedo Blows Them Up."[53]

What Dipper and his accomplices encountered that night can be explained by a patent in the U.S. Patent and Trademark Office. After the Harrison Horror, Philip K. Clover—an artist and inventor from Ohio—filed a patent called "Improvement in Coffin-Torpedoes." Its purpose was to, in Clover's words:

> Provide a means which shall successfully prevent the unauthorized resurrection of dead bodies; and with this end in view my invention consists of a peculiarly-constructed torpedo, adapted to be readily secured to the coffin and the body of the contained corpse in such manner that any attempt to remove the body after burial will cause the discharge of the cartridge contained in the torpedo and injury or death of the desecrator of the grave.[54]

Clover's device was essentially a metal pipe filled with gunpowder and balls, wired to the body, such as the arms or legs. It was placed at the head of the coffin, aimed squarely where body snatchers were most likely to break in, and loaded just before closing the coffin. When opened, the device discharged its contents with "deadly force," which one newspaper at the time jokingly wrote was "guaranteed to blow a body-snatcher over the highest church steeple."[55] The device was never intended to be permanent. The patent mentioned that it was not waterproof but would be "preserved in effective condition until such time as the body would be of no use to robbers."[56] Depending on the weather, only a little over a week was needed for a body to fully decompose.

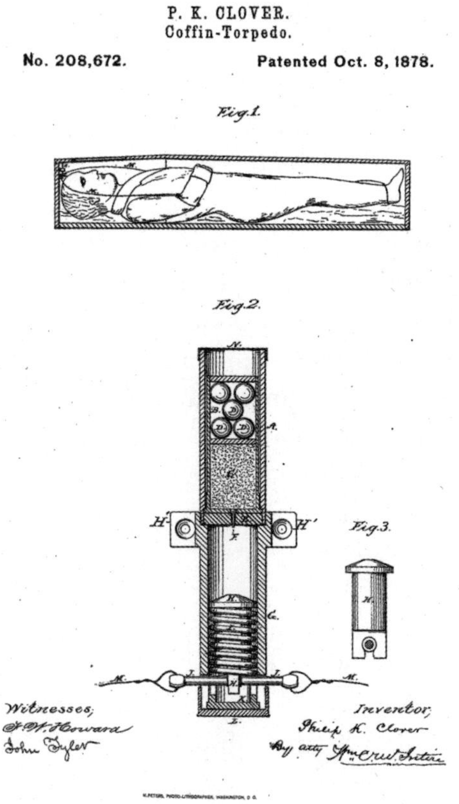

In the 19th century the word "torpedo" referred to weapons that functioned like landmines. The "weapons that wait," as they were called, were first used in warfare by the Confederacy in the American Civil War, and only in the 20th century did the term "torpedo" become associated with naval warfare. Clover's device actually functioned more like a shotgun, but Thomas N. Howell, a former probate judge also from Ohio, filed a patent for a "Grave-Torpedo" a year after Clover in 1879, which functioned like a landmine.[57]

Philip K. Clover's "coffin torpedo" functioned similarly to a shotgun. (United States Patent and Trademark Office)

Howell's device was wired to the coffin, and placed above it in the dirt instead of inside, and if triggered would cause the "dirt to be thrown in all directions, and injuring, if not killing, the would-be graverobbers."[58] As a method of protecting the dead, it was a double-edged sword: if triggered, the resulting explosion stopped the body snatchers, but it also damaged the body inside the coffin: "It would seem, however, that this invention is intended to have a moral, rather than a practical effect, for it is difficult to see how it can explode without demolishing the dead body," as a Virginia newspaper observed at the time.[59] Howell later patented an improved version of his torpedo that was designed to minimize "all danger of premature explosion or disarrangement of the mechanism while charging the torpedo and adjusting it in position."[60]

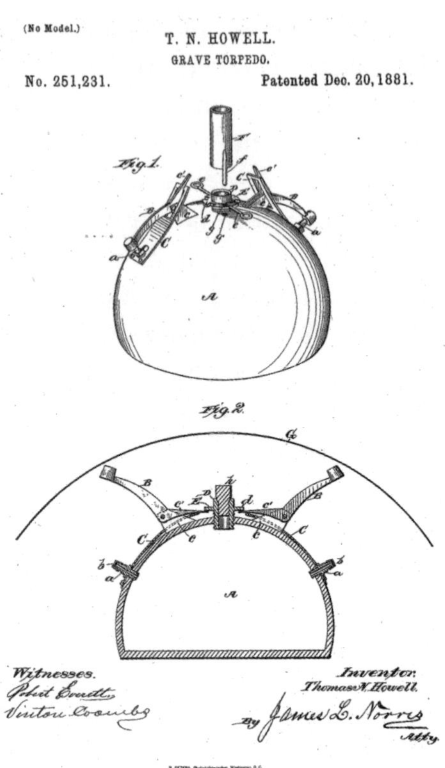

Thomas N. Howell's "grave torpedo" functioned more like a landmine. (United States Patent and Trademark Office)

Coffin torpedoes were used not just to prevent body snatching, but also grave robbery. The grave of Mrs. William C. Whitney, a wealthy woman buried in New York, contained valuable jewels, and to protect them was "sown with powerful torpedoes. The coffin is hemmed about with them, and the ghoul who undertook to strike his spade beneath the surface would invite swift destruction…There is no secret about the torpedoes. All the village talks of them."[61] Other defenses were used to prevent bodies from being held for ransom. Abraham Lincoln's corpse was almost stolen from Oak Ridge Cemetery in Springfield, Illinois, in 1876, 11 years after his assassination. Crime boss "Big Jim" Kennally, an Irish immigrant who led a gang of counterfeiters, schemed to ransom Lincoln's corpse for the release of his partner in crime Benjamin Boyd from prison, and 2,000 dollars cash. But the group needed someone with expertise in grave robbing to carry out their plan, and hired a man named Lewis Swegles to assist them.

Lincoln's aboveground tomb in Oak Ridge Cemetery was surprisingly undefended: a single padlocked door was all that stood in their way.[62] On November 7, 1876, election night, when they correctly assumed that most people would be distracted, two of Kennally's gang and Swegles made their way to Lincoln's tomb, cut through the padlock, and broke open Lincoln's sarcophagus. Swegles then left to retrieve the wagon to load the body and escape, but there was no wagon: Swegles was an informant for the Secret Service.[63] The Secret Service had been established the same day Lincoln was assassinated, not to protect the president as it does today, but to go after people who counterfeited money like Kennally and Boyd.

Swegles gave the signal to the waiting Secret Service members and Pinkerton agents they hired to assist them to arrest the grave robbers, but one of the Secret Service member's guns went off by accident, and the thieves fled. In the confusion, and in the dark, the Pinkertons and Secret Service members shot at each other, thinking the grave robbers were attacking them. No one was injured, but Kennally's gang got away. They were later arrested and served a year in prison.[64] For years Lincoln was buried in an unmarked grave in the tomb's basement for his safety, until he was moved into a vault in the tomb in 1887, but it wasn't until his tomb finished being rebuilt in 1901 that he was finally laid to rest for good in a truly impenetrable place: a 10-foot-deep vault, inside a steel cage, that was then filled with concrete, where he rests today.[65] The Secret Service took on the protection of presidents after the assassination of President William McKinley in 1901.

The burial safe and burial vault were also introduced as a result of the Harrison Horror, versions of which were patented by Andrew Van Bibber and George W. Boyd in 1878 and 1879 respectively. Like Clover and Howell, both were Ohioans—the state where the Harrison Horror occurred.[66] Bibber described the purpose of his burial safe:

> [To] provide a strong and secure protecting-case for coffins, which, when placed within a grave and properly fastened and weighted, shall prevent access to the coffin for the purpose of removing the corpse therefrom within the time necessary for body-stealers to perform their work. To this end the invention consists in a case much larger than the coffin, composed of wrought-iron or steel, preferably in the form of bars, and provided with a suitable cover adapted to be locked or otherwise secured on the inside of the case.[67]

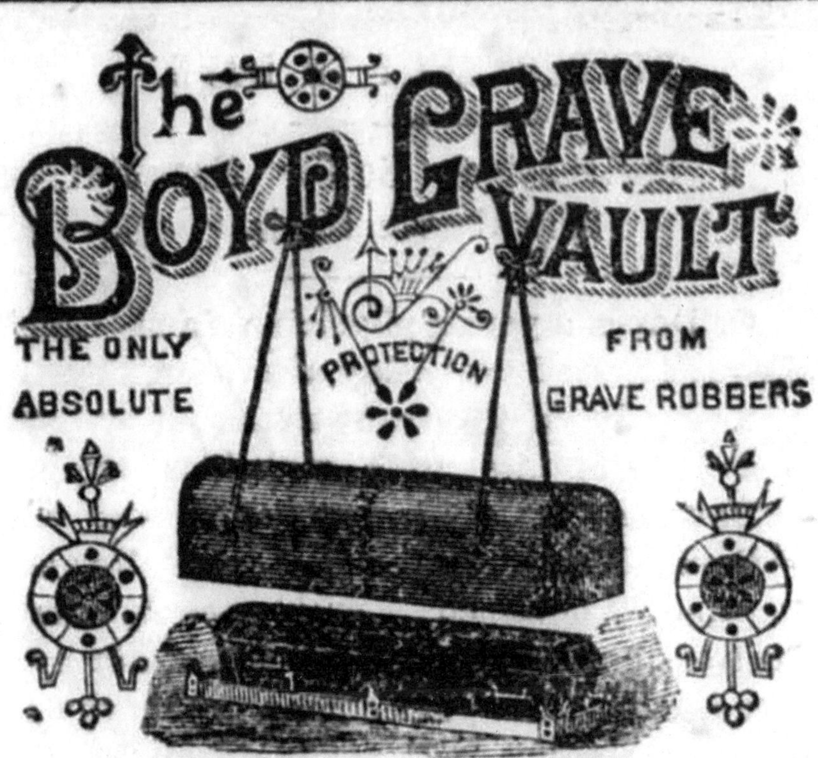

No community is safe from the grave robber. So protect your dead by using a BOYD GRAVE VAULT. It is self-locking; keeps out Vermin as well as Burglars. For sale by all undertakers. Manufactured by Springfield Manufacturing Company, Springfield, O. Branch office with

FLANNER & HOMMOWN,

72 North Illinois Street,

INDIANAPOLIS, IND.

Advertisement for the Boyd Grave Vault. (Library of Congress)

It was essentially a mortsafe, or a cage, but one that didn't cover the top of the grave, but the coffin itself inside the grave.[68] The cage was larger than the coffin so that, as the grave was filled, the dirt would go through its bars and weigh it down so it couldn't be pulled out, and to hinder access to the padlocks that secured it.[69] Unless body snatchers knew about the defense in advance, they likely wouldn't have the tools to break through in a timely fashion.

Unlike Bibber's, Boyd's burial case was not a cage, but a "burglar-proof" metal vault that enclosed the coffin, which consisted of two metal pieces—the bottom and the cover—that were secured together with spring-catches, designed to be impossible to open once closed. Another difference with Bibber's invention was that it was designed to not be overly expensive, so that it could be "purchased by persons of limited means."[70] Similar inventions were marketed for their effectiveness in preventing body snatching: "Protect your dead by using the Okey Burial Vault. The only positively and continuously air and water tight, burglar proof, indestructible and reliably sanitary burial vault manufactured."[71] A man in Nashville planned to bury himself in a sarcophagus of his own design to thwart body snatchers active in the area.[72]

These patents reflected an awareness of body-snatchers' methods, which became more well known after scandals like Harrison's. One patent, which strapped the person in the coffin so they couldn't be pulled out by the neck—similar to the coffin collar, which strapped bodies in the coffin by the neck with a metal collar, which was only known to have been used in Scotland—noted:

> The nature and utility of my invention may be the better understood, the mode of operation practiced by "body-snatchers" or "resurrectionists" may be briefly explained as follows: The operators, having reached the grave and ascertained the point exactly above the head of the corpse, employ a post-hole digger, or similar implement, first sinking it into, and then drawing it up with, the earth until the coffin is reached. A large hole is thus cut in the earth immediately over the head of the corpse. The coffin-lid is then battered open, and the subject drawn to the surface by means of a hook placed under the chin.[73]

Aside from a handful of cases reported in newspapers, there is little evidence that coffin torpedoes were widely used.[74] One barrier was that they were too expensive for the vast majority of people, according to a Pennsylvania newspaper: "Burglar alarms, savage dogs, armed watchmen, telegraph lines, gongs...are now employed in the various Philadelphia cemeteries to keep in the ground the remains of rich people."[75] They were also wildly impractical. Why go to so much trouble for something that wouldn't be a problem after a week when the body had fully decomposed? Why not use any other number of defenses that didn't involve deadly weapons? The *New-York Tribune* summarized the absurdity of the coffin torpedo in 1896:

> It is a grewsome and utterly senseless ingenuity that thus reaches into the sepulchre, making posthumous needs for the poor child of mortality slumbering there. Some of them may be real enough, but most of them are probably fanciful, and intended to act in a money-making way on the sentiment and apprehension of survivors. There are enough devices of the sort already without any new rush of invention into that dismal field, and if it be said of the coffin torpedo, the latest of them, that it fills a long-felt want, the remark is also in order that the want is an unreasonable one. A system of bombshells planted in graveyards does not seem to be a necessary protective expedient, and it would expend most of its effect upon posterity, who always sooner or later want the premises for other use.[76]

The coffin torpedo was an attempt to profit from the fear of the body snatchers after the Harrison Horror, like any other number of inventions that failed to catch on and become commercially successful. In the annals of American patents, it takes a prominent place alongside other patents that used excessive force to solve a problem, such as the gun-powered mousetrap from 1882, which was what it sounded like: a mousetrap with a handgun attached pointed squarely where the mouse would trigger it. Around the same time that deadly devices were being invented to prevent body snatching, a very different solution was proposed to prevent body snatching: cremation. If there was no body to bury, there was no body to snatch, perhaps the only truly foolproof method to avoid being untimely resurrected.

★ ★ ★

Before Philip Syng Physick died in 1837, the University of Pennsylvania's professor of anatomy in the early 19th century left unusual instructions for his final disposition. Physick's successor at the university,

William E. Horner, later bemoaned that his instructions led "the public to infer that no place nor person was too sacred for the anatomist," and could only be explained by "sensitiveness, we may perhaps say obliquity, produced by long-continued retirement and indisposition."[77] Despite having dissected countless people, when it came to his own mortal remains, Physick avoided the scalpel at all costs.

Physick requested, first, that his body be left in his home to putrefy, to render it useless for dissection. Second, he was to be placed in a wooden coffin, inside a lead coffin, which was to be soldered.[78] Third, a watchman was to preside over his grave every night for six weeks after he was interred at Christ Church Burial Ground in Old City. By one account, Physick's fears came from personal experience. After Dr. Benjamin Rush—a founding father and prominent physician—passed away in 1813, a body snatcher was said to have approached Physick at his home and asked if he wanted Rush's body for 20 dollars, and that he could deliver it to the university the next day.[79] Physick refused the offer. Both Rush's and Physick's graves can be visited in Christ Church Burial Ground today, but while we can be reasonably certain that Physick still rests in peace, it's an open question if the same is true of Rush, if the story is to be believed.

Many self-styled "enlightened" physicians contrasted themselves with the so-called "superstitious" public, and made the argument that because the body was just matter, people should have no qualms with their bodies being dissected after death. The idea that the dead are just matter can be traced back to the Greek philosopher Diogenes, and it is empirically true: biologically and even in most belief systems, the body cannot feel pain after death. But it is an idea that has historically not been widely accepted.[80] Many people believe that a corpse should be treated with respect and not used for other purposes, whether their beliefs are informed by religion or simply a feeling of squeamishness or superstition about one's remains being tampered with.

Judged by how they disposed of their own bodies, physicians' views seemed broadly similar to most at the time. For most anatomists, the idea that the body was "mere matter" extended to the poor, but not to their own bodies.

An 1879 issue of *Penn Monthly* noted, "I am aware that there have been men…who have voluntarily willed their bodies to be dissected, but they have been extremely few, and their heartless wish has not aroused the admiration of any considerable number of people."[81] Like most others at the time, physicians rarely donated their bodies to dissection, and actively avoided being dissected. It was a double standard that the *Philadelphia Inquirer* poked fun at in 1878:

> The profession itself should be above the superstitious and sentimental prejudices which ordinary mortals entertain regarding the disposition of their bodies, and should be sufficiently interested in the advancement of science to devote their remains to this holy cause. Let every physician, then, at once make a will devoting his body to the dissecting room of any college he may prefer, and there will be no further need of grave robbing.[82]

"The Surgeon's Warning" by English poet Robert Southey perfectly encapsulates the anxiety of physicians like Physick over their remains. The poem is about a dying surgeon trying to avoid being dissected after his death:

> Bury me in lead when I am dead,
> My brethren I intreat,
> And see the coffin weigh'd I beg
> Lest the Plumber should be a cheat.
>
> And let it be solder'd closely down
> Strong as strong can be I implore,
> And put it in a patent coffin,
> That I may rise no more.
>
> If they carry me off in the patent coffin
> Their labour will be in vain,
> Let the Undertaker see it bought of the maker
> Who lives by St. Martin's lane.
>
> And bury me in my brother's church
> For that will safer be,
> And I implore lock the church door
> And pray take care of the key.
>
> And all night long let three stout men
> The vestry watch within,
> To each man give a gallon of beer
> And a keg of Holland's gin;

Powder and ball and blunder-buss
To save me if he can,
And eke five guineas if he shoot
A resurrection man.

And let them watch me for three weeks
My wretched corpse to save,
For then I think that I may stink
Enough to rest in my grave.

The surgeon did not rest peacefully, and was dissected by his own students:

So they carried the sack a-pick-a-back
And they carv'd him bone from bone,
But what became of the Surgeon's soul
Was never to mortal known.[83]

However, there were exceptions to this near-universal aversion to dissection. In his will, John Collins Warren, professor of anatomy and surgery at Harvard Medical School, stipulated:

> The final and principal object of writing this letter is this, which regards the disposition of my mortal remains after the spirit has quitted them.
>
> 1. Let the body be injected with arsenic after death, *soon* [to preserve it]...
>
> [...]
>
> 3. The body afterwards to be removed to the Medical College; examined or dissected according to circumstances. Any morbid parts to be carefully preserved; and particular attention is to be paid to the heart, spleen and prostate gland.
>
> 4. The bones to be carefully preserved, whitened, articulated, and placed in the lecture room of the Medical College, near my bust; affording, as I hope, a lesson useful, at the same time, to morality and science.
>
> I earnestly request that you and my family will lay aside any natural feeling of opposition to this my last request; considering that it is for the interest of humanity and for mine and their honor.[84]

Warren's instructions were followed to the letter, and today his skeleton is housed in the Warren Anatomical Museum, but it is not publicly displayed.

While physicians weren't the first to volunteer their bodies for dissection, they were among the first to endorse cremation in the modern era, a then-radical method of disposing of the dead.[85] Cremation was of course an ancient practice, but one that went out of favor in the

West after the rise of Christianity.[86] While some Native Americans practiced cremation, in 19th-century America it was widely considered blasphemous. This was a time when it was believed that the body had to be buried whole to be resurrected before the Last Judgment. Gradually, the belief in the necessity of keeping the body intact in the grave gave way to an acceptance of the idea that even a cremated body could be resurrected by an omnipotent God. Before cremation became common, the American Medical Association came close to publicly endorsing cremation in 1866.[87] One person who helped introduce "modern" cremation to America was the Pennsylvania physician Francis Julius LeMoyne, a graduate of Jefferson Medical College.

In Washington, Pennsylvania—a suburb of Pittsburgh from where LeMoyne came—he built the first American crematory in 1876. It still stands there today, on a site known by locals as "Gallows Hill," which was formerly used for executions. LeMoyne's house also still stands in Washington, Pennsylvania, which was a stop on the Underground

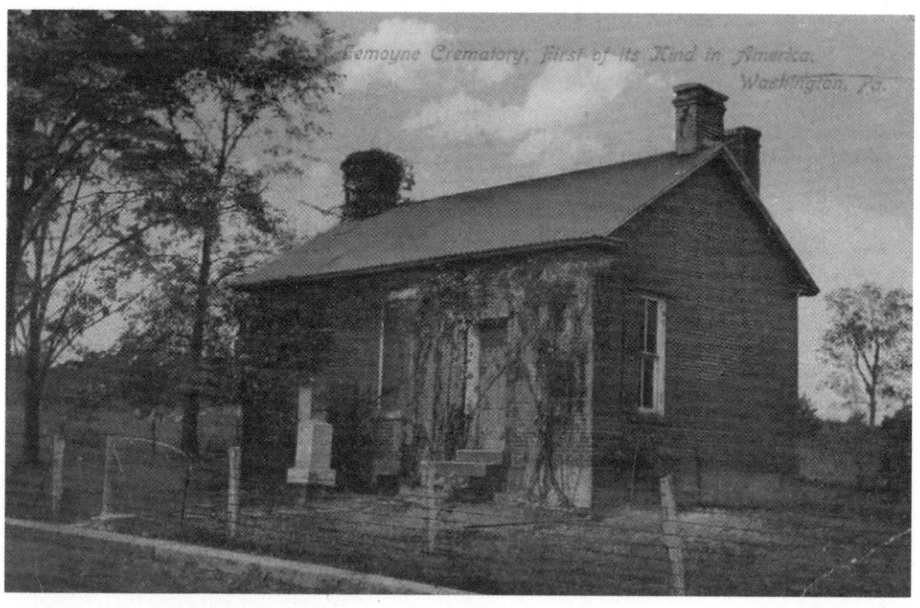

Lemoyne Crematory, First of its Kind in America.
Washington, Pa.

LeMoyne Crematory, America's first crematory in Washington, Pennsylvania, established in 1876. (Wikimedia Commons)

Railroad; LeMoyne was an abolitionist and a cremationist. One of LeMoyne's arguments supporting cremation was that cremation was more sanitary than burial, that dead bodies contaminated the soil and groundwater and spread disease. Another was overcrowding of the dead in cities like Philadelphia. Cemeteries were relocated as the city expanded; they're not as permanent as one generally thinks, and Philadelphia as we know it today is strewn with former cemeteries beneath its buildings. Cremation is an ancient practice, and LeMoyne and other supporters were attempting to turn it into a modern death rite on a scientific basis; however, the miasma theory of disease, which held that "bad" air emanating from rotting matter, including the dead, spreads disease, was later debunked by the germ theory of disease in the late 19th century.

While not the most prominent argument, cremationists also cited body snatching to support cremation. In 1882, *The Philadelphia Inquirer* suggested:

> What can be said now in favor of converting into ashes the human body, from which life has fled, has already been said over and over again, but the recent disclosure of cupidity and moral disregard of everything that the majority of the race have been taught to consider most sacred illustrates anew how uncertain is the security of the repose of the dead even when the most careful precautions are taken to attain that end.[88]

In 1891 the same paper remarked, "Cremating of the dead seems to be the only thing that will do away with the grave robber's occupation."[89] *The Urn*, a pro-cremation publication, frequently wrote about body snatching, such as roundups of recent incidents with the headline "Graves Robbed and Desecrated," or noting:

> It seems almost a pity to disturb the illusive dream that cemeteries are sleeping places of the dead as the name implies, yet it is a pathetic fact that neither the body of the pauper, buried without a tear, that of the millionaire committed to the vault with more than royal magnificence, nor even that of a martyred president, placed in a tomb protected by bolts and bars, is safe from the sacrilegious hand of the resurrectionist...The burying of the dead has manifold disadvantages, but the Christian world is not yet ready to hasten the workings of nature by burning the dead...[body snatching] must lead the thoughtful to think seriously of the advantages of the cremating process over that of burial.[90]

An American physician wrote in an 1887 book that with cremation, "The darkness and the dampness of the earth have been escaped, and so have the perils of grave-snatching, the indecencies of a possible dissecting-room, and the nameless horrors of putrefaction."[91] Grave robbing was also cited, such as the attempted theft and ransom of Lincoln.

The "first" cremation in America in LeMoyne's crematory was Baron Joseph Henry Louis Charles de Palm, a destitute Bavarian nobleman who immigrated to the United States, who wanted to be cremated not out of fear of body snatching, but fear of premature burial.[92] Taphophobia—the fear of accidentally being buried alive—was not unreasonable given that vital signs could be so faint as to be imperceptible to doctors of the time, such as someone's pulse or breathing, especially if they were comatose, sedated, or suffering from other conditions. Still, such cases were exceedingly rare, and in the 18th and 19th centuries the fear of premature burial was disproportionate to how often it actually occurred.

George Washington's last words were, "Have me decently buried; and do not let my body be put into the vault in less than three days after I am dead," to ensure he was not prematurely buried, and when his secretary confirmed he understood, Washington's last words were "Tis well."[93] In 1913, a cotton broker in Philadelphia, Andrew J. Turner, died. His death was newsworthy because of an odd request he made to his wife before he died: to not be buried for two weeks after his death, to ensure that he would not be buried alive.[94] After his younger brother died three years prior, Turner had a dream of "his brother clawing at the lid of his coffin," and he had been afraid he would suffer the same fate ever since.[95] His wife honored his wishes. In Williamsport, Pennsylvania in 1891, a man built a tomb to ensure that none of his relatives would ever face the fate of premature burial. It had five compartments for five people:

> [The compartments are] lined with heavy felt to prevent injury, should the supposed dead recover and become panic-stricken. Ducts supply fresh air to all compartments so that one in a state of trance may not be suffocated. No person, other than the holders of the keys, can unlock and open the massive iron compartment covers from the outside, but they can be opened from the inside by handwheels.[96]

"Safety" coffins were even developed to prevent premature burial. A wire inside the coffin was attached to a bell that, if the person buried suddenly came to, they could ring and call for help. There was also of course a means for fresh air to circulate in the coffin so that the person could breathe in the meantime. Some claim that the phrases "saved by the bell" and "dead ringers" come from this practice, but the terms likely came well after the invention of the safety coffin. There is no evidence that safety coffins were actually used or saved anyone's life. But patents for various safety coffins, like the coffin torpedo, reflect a widespread fear that entrepreneurs tried to capitalize on.

The cremation of Baron de Palm in 1876 was widely covered by the press, and was highly controversial. LeMoyne died three years after he built his crematory in 1879, and practicing what he preached, was also cremated there. Other physicians followed LeMoyne's lead in being cremated. Samuel D. Gross, professor of surgery at Jefferson Medical College, made national news in 1884 for his decision to be cremated in LeMoyne's crematory. Gross wrote in his autobiography, "A man who spends much of his time in the dissecting-room, and looks at the horrible features of the putrefying bodies as they lie before him upon the tables, is not likely to hesitate between burial and cremation."[97] The experience of dissection was one reason physicians were early adopters of cremation, but were also persuaded by scientific and practical arguments for cremation. Cremation gradually became accepted as an alternative to burial in the 20th century; the Catholic Church lifted its ban on cremation in 1963. Today over 50 percent of Americans are cremated after death, not because of the possibility of body snatching, but in part because it's more affordable.

★ ★ ★

The coffin torpedo, burial safe, and burial vault came near the end of the era of body snatchers in America, when they would no longer be needed after laws were put in place to regulate the bodies medical schools were allowed to dissect.[98] The most logical way to stop body snatching wasn't a torpedo, but legislation. Throughout the 19th century, laws were put in place to punish body snatchers, but the Ohio Anatomy Law of 1881, passed as a result of the Harrison Horror, was one of many laws passed in the late 19th century to address the supply problems that actually caused body snatching. Pennsylvania's anatomy law would lead the way to legislation that finally ended the era of the body snatchers. But how did such laws work? Why did it take over a century and a half for most states to address the root causes of body snatching, when it had already been addressed in the United Kingdom as early as 1832? What happened to body snatchers if they got caught? How were they punished under the law, and how were they punished when caught by everyday people, who meted out their own vigilante justice?

CHAPTER 6

"A Resurrectionist Punished"

Body Snatching and the Law

> The law does not prevent our obtaining the body of an individual if we think proper; for there is no person, let his situation in life be what it may, whom, if I were disposed to dissect, I could not obtain...The law only enhances the price, and does not prevent the exhumation; nobody is secured by the law, it only adds to the price of the subject.
>
> —SIR ASTLEY COOPER, BRITISH SURGEON AND ANATOMIST[1]

In 1857 William J. McKnight was 21 years old and in his first year practicing medicine in Brookville, Pennsylvania, northeast of Pittsburgh. He was a "pioneer" physician who rode on horseback to visit his patients through "rain, mud, sleet, cold, snow, and darkness"; before daily mail, neighbors of the sick travelled on foot or horseback to call on him.[2] Life in the country was generally healthier than in cities like Philadelphia, where population and trade growth increased the spread of disease, but wherever one lived, medical treatments weren't much different from the previous century.[3] While bloodletting fell out of favor in Brookville around 1850, the medicines of the day also had dubious value.[4]

From the mid- to late 19th century, two ancient theories of the cause of disease—an imbalance of "humors" in the body (blood, phlegm, yellow bile, and black bile), and "miasma," (bad air) from decomposing matter—were disproven by germ theory. As we know today, diseases are actually transmitted through pathogenic microorganisms that can only be seen with the aid of a microscope. As the understanding of the human body improved through dissection, so did medicine, but bodies were hard to come by in rural Pennsylvania.

When a resident near Brookville died, the area's five physicians became pioneer resurrectionists. Henry Southerland was described by McKnight as "a stout, perfect specimen of physical manhood" who could "drink, swear, wrestle, shoot, jump…and raft."[5] A 30-year-old Black man with a wife and child, his father was said to have "held General Washington's horse at the laying of the corner-stone of the national capitol at Washington" before he escaped slavery in Virginia and settled in Pennsylvania.[6] The idea to dissect Henry after he died of a fever was J. G. Simons's, a local doctor and aspiring surgeon who believed it was a "good chance for a subject and a surgical school to advance himself and assist the rest of us."[7] Henry wasn't the first. In the winter of 1854/55, the body of an Irishman who froze to death in Clarion County was snatched and dissected in Brookville.[8]

The five doctors and two "medically inclined" accomplices—K. L. Blood and Augustus Bell—met in Blood's drug store, appropriately enough, on the night of October 31, "All Hallows' Eve" as it was known then.[9] After some drank whiskey, they made their way to the graveyard. McKnight and another stood watch while their companions vigorously shoveled the earth from the grave, broke open the coffin lid, pulled Henry's body out with a rope, left his clothes behind, and filled the grave. They transported the body to Dr. Clark's vacant house and parted ways for the night. Their plans for a secret anatomy class there were cut short after one of the doctors talked, and word soon spread of their crime. Fearing for Dr. Clark, they moved Henry's body to Blood's ice-house (a building used to store ice before refrigerators were invented) in a coffee sack. The physicians then committed a shocking act of mutilation: they skinned Henry's body and removed his fingers and toes to "prevent identification and for our personal safety," in McKnight's words.[10]

With Brookville on high alert, the group schemed to get Henry's body out of town, but their attempt to avoid getting caught led to exactly that. A doctor from a neighboring town agreed to take the body and transport it in his wagon, but their plan broke down when Dr. A. P. Heichhold, who was responsible for unlocking the door, lost the ice-house key, and went to search for something to force the door open. McKnight and Dr. John Dowling then arrived to help load the body in the wagon but soon left because they were told not to linger if the door was still locked, to avoid drawing attention. The wagon came, but with the door locked and no one present, the doctor continued on his way. Finally, Dr. Heichhold found a hatchet, broke open the ice-house door, and departed once his part of the job was complete.

The next day McKnight and Dowling went to confirm that Henry's body had been removed, and just as they discovered that their plan had failed disastrously, a young boy walked by who noticed them and the ice-house's broken lock. When McKnight and Dowling realized they were being watched, they fled, and the boy walked into the horrifying scene inside: a body with its "breast sawed open, the bowels and entrails removed, the toe- and finger-nails cut off at the first joint, and the skin of the entire body removed."[11] The boy ran and told everyone he passed what he found, and locals converged on the building. It was soon surmised why the body was there and whom it belonged to, and a throng of people went to Henry's grave and confirmed that it was empty. Other recently dug graves in the cemetery were opened, but no other bodies were missing. Some still hired watchmen to guard them.

Pennsylvania Congressman David Barclay, a lawyer, took charge of the prosecution, who had it out for K. L. Blood and McKnight for political reasons. On the advice of his brother, also a lawyer, McKnight preempted Barclay's charges and turned himself in. He paid a fine of 25 dollars and fees and served no jail time. Barclay indicted Blood and McKnight, but McKnight couldn't be punished for the same crime twice. The result of Blood's prosecution has been lost to history. Of the affair, a local newspaper commented:

> Taking everything into consideration, it was one of the most inhuman and barbarous acts ever committed in a civilized community; and although the instigators and perpetrators may escape the punishment which their brutality demands, they cannot fail to receive the indignant frowns of an insulted community. They may evade a prosecution through the technicalities of the law, and they may laugh it off, and when we have no assurance but that our bodies, or those of our friends, may be treated in the same manner, cold and hardened must be the wretch who does not feel the flame of indignation rise in his breast at the perpetration of such an offence.[12]

McKnight, who would later go on to become a state senator, published an account of these events in 1897 in the local newspaper with the racist headline "Brookville's Pioneer Resurrection or 'Who Skinned the N_____.' The Truth Told for the First Time, by the Only One Now Living of the Seven Who Were Engaged in it." At the time of the events and well after, McKnight felt little or no remorse for his actions, which demonstrated how the use of Black bodies for dissection was normalized in the 19th century, supported by racist ideas. Bodies for dissection were scarce in Brookville, as they were in other rural parts of Pennsylvania, but even in dense cities like Philadelphia anatomists struggled to supply their schools. McKnight's story shows how far some were willing to go in pursuit of medical careers and medical progress, and how they came up against state laws that were passed as awareness of the practice spread.

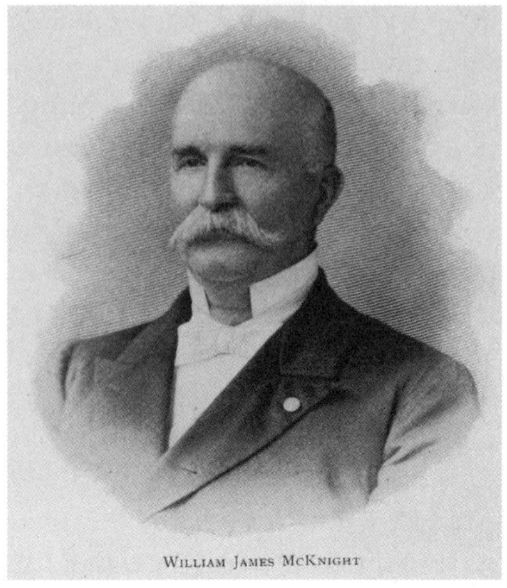

William J. McKnight, convicted body snatcher, later a Pennsylvania state senator. (Internet Archive)

For a crime some believed to be worse than murder, it might come as a surprise that body snatching was only a misdemeanor. American courts followed the precedent set by the British case of Rex v. Lynn in 1788. The ruling held that body snatching wasn't a felony because dead bodies aren't property, which is still true today.[13] Many states had no laws against body snatching well into the 19th century. When caught, body snatchers were charged with other crimes. Stealing a cadaver's clothing was a felony, which is why resurrectionists were careful to leave them behind in the coffin. Some were not so cautious.

The D.C. body-snatcher George Christian's clothing was always "taken from the grave; he, therefore, was usually well dressed."[14] At a time when no law was on the books for body snatching in D.C., the resurrectionist William M. Jansen was charged under a health regulation that prevented bodies from being transported on city streets without a permit.[15]

Others were indicted for trespassing or any other number of violations. Before the American Revolution, body snatchers in Pennsylvania and other colonies were also charged under a 1604 English act that prohibited digging up a body for the purposes of witchcraft.[16]

Until well into the 20th century, the vast majority of people would have never desired to donate their body to science, but even if they wanted to, it wasn't legal to sell your own body because you technically didn't own it. Still, that didn't stop some from trying and even succeeding in selling their own bodies to medical colleges before their death. In 1887 a man named Stamper who died near Newark, New York, sold his body to either a medical student or the college he studied in, six months before his death, to pay for whiskey.[17] His body was discovered during shipment, but after learning of its destination and the student's explanation, the local coroner let it go on its way. Charley Keaton, the assistant of body-snatcher William Cunningham in Ohio, sold his body to Ohio Medical College, as Cunningham did. According to the *Cincinnati Enquirer*:

> Indeed, he seemed rather to prefer that his skeleton should stand beside that of old "Cunny" in the museum of the College than to molder to nothingness in the dark, damp earth, and in life he frequently contemplated Cunny's skeleton as it stands, spade in hand, in the College, evidently reflecting that he would some day stand beside it, and keep the "old man" company through the many years that the college shall stand, instead of being consigned to the changes and final nothingness of the Potter's Field grave.[18]

While even today no one owns a person's body after they die, the body has quasi-property rights: the wishes of the deceased, such as how they want to dispose of their body, or the wishes of the family must be respected. While one can donate their body to medical schools today, they still can't sell it.

The first American law that prohibited body snatching passed in New York in 1789 in response to an anatomy riot the previous year. The law made the act punishable by fine, incarceration, or the pillory—a device that locked one's head and hands in holes and subjected them to public humiliation—or other forms of corporal punishment.[19] The use of the pillory as punishment was outlawed in the United States in 1839, although it was not abolished in Delaware until 1905.[20] Judges could impose a fine of any amount or jail time of any length, or none at all.[21]

In 1796 New Hampshire made body snatching punishable by no more than 1,000 dollars, no more than one year in prison, or a public whipping, all at the judge's discretion; Vermont passed a similar law in 1804.[22] In 1815 Massachusetts, and in 1817 Connecticut, made body snatching and possession of stolen dead bodies punishable by 1,000 dollars and a year in prison; body snatchers and the doctors who received their bodies were equally liable.[23] All other states in New England had similar laws against body snatching by 1818.[24] In 1819 New York increased the penalty for body snatching to five years in prison.[25] Corporal punishment—more medieval methods of punishment such as the pillory—gradually faded from use, as well as punishment for possession of dead bodies, which protected doctors from legal liability.[26] In 1831 Ohio made body snatching punishable by up to a 1,000-dollar fine or a month in jail.[27]

Compared with other states, Pennsylvania was late in criminalizing body snatching. The state prohibited the practice in 1849, when the state legislature passed "An Act…For the Protection of Cemeteries and Grave Yards." According to the act:

> Any person who shall willfully…open any tomb or grave…and clandestinely remove or attempt to remove any body or remains therefrom, shall be guilty of a misdemeanor, and shall, upon conviction thereof, before any justice of the peace of the county where the said offence is committed, be punished by a fine, at the discretion of the justice, according to the aggravation of the offence, of not less than one or more than fifty dollars…and by imprisonment, according to the aggravation of the offence, at the discretion of the court, for a term not exceeding one year.[28]

In the 1855 "Act To Protect Burial Grounds," the penalty was increased to a minimum of 100 dollars and one to three years in prison.[29] Given that McKnight paid a quarter of the minimum fine and served no jail time, the judge clearly let him off easy. According to John Collins Warren, professor of anatomy and surgery at Harvard Medical School:

> Two or three times, our agents were actually seized by the police, and recognized to appear in court. One or two were brought in guilty, and punished by fine;

> but the law officers, being more liberal in their views than the city officers [in New York], made the penalty as small as possible.[30]

In some states judges had the power to give body snatchers a slap on the wrist, or if public pressure was great, a harsher sentence. Laws didn't deter body snatchers: the trade was so lucrative, to many it was worth the risk. The doctors they supplied often paid their legal fees and even supported their families while they served prison time.[31] When the body of former Congressman John Scott Harrison was snatched and the Ohio Medical College's janitor was arrested for concealing the body, faculty posted his bail—a whopping 5,000 dollars—which further inflamed the public's anger against the college.[32] To protect themselves, in other highly public cases anatomists denied that they had made arrangements with body snatchers who were caught, and refused to post bail to not give the appearance that they were engaged in the trade.

When caught, some body snatchers found creative ways to evade the law. Charles O. Morton was arrested with two accomplices in Toledo, Ohio, for snatching and shipping bodies to Ann Arbor, Michigan in 1878.[33] After his arrest Morton said he felt sick, and his body was found to be covered with eruptions, which physicians believed was smallpox. Morton was quarantined in the "pest-house," where he escaped and was never found. It was believed he rubbed his body with croton oil, which is highly toxic to humans, to fake his illness. William Cunningham, the Ohio body snatcher, once got away with stealing two bodies twice.[34] Cunningham and his assistants were arrested while transporting two bodies they resurrected, which were sent to a funeral home. After they made bail, someone who claimed to be from the coroner's office contacted the undertaker to release the cadavers into his care. It turned out the coroner's office had never contacted the funeral home: the body snatchers had taken back the bodies. Without the bodies, there was no evidence to charge them with a crime, and the police dropped the charges. Cunningham was also once caught body snatching in a graveyard by locals, but as he was being transported from the cemetery for his arrest, he convinced the men to stop at the saloon.[35] After a few drinks, they decided to let him go, but instead of giving up for the night Cunningham went back to the cemetery to finish the job with his accomplices.

Some Southern universities forced enslaved African Americans to perform body snatching for them; legally considered property themselves, they couldn't be arrested for body snatching.[36] The Medical College of Georgia had five "resurrection slaves" around the mid-19th century, but the job rested solely with Grandison Harris in 1852, when he was purchased by the college in Charleston, South Carolina.[37] After the Civil War, Harris became an employee of the college and performed the same tasks. Chris Baker was born into slavery in the Medical College of Virginia where his parents worked, and he also stole bodies for them.[38]

Body snatchers were at risk of legal and extra-legal punishment, or vigilante justice, when everyday people took the law into their own hands. In 1834 a Virginia student who attempted to take the body of an enslaved Black man buried on a farmer's property was shot in the back; the student, who recovered from his injury, complained to the authorities, but they declined to prosecute the farmer.[39] In Albany, New York in 1859 a body snatcher caught in the act by the inhabitants of a nearby porter-house was given the choice of prosecution or 100 lashes on his bare back with a rawhide whip.[40] He chose the whip, and a newspaper reported that the man "submitted to the infliction like a martyr, not making any outcry. Having received the punishment, he resumed his garments and started off in the direction of Schenectady."[41]

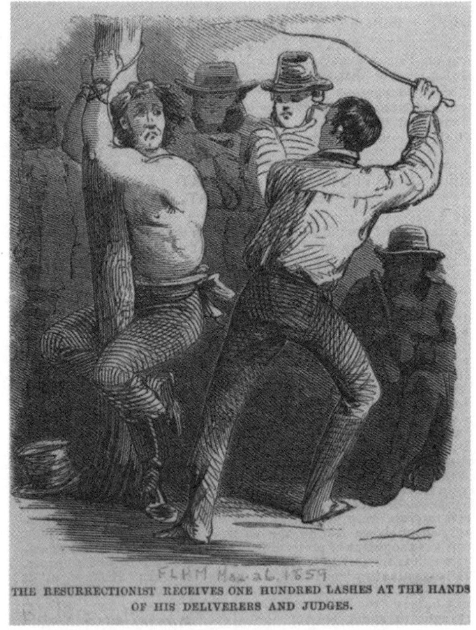
THE RESURRECTIONIST RECEIVES ONE HUNDRED LASHES AT THE HANDS OF HIS DELIVERERS AND JUDGES.

Bellew (also featured on the cover of this book) received his punishment for body snatching. (The New York Public Library)

Doctors were vulnerable after they received stolen bodies but before they destroyed the evidence through dissection. When body snatching was suspected, the police might search the college, or mobs might descend on anatomists' homes or medical schools, bent on destruction and violence. Some schools even relocated or closed their doors due to riots. Philadelphia was the site of America's first anatomy, or resurrection, riot in 1765, when William Shippen Jr. fled his home from the "sailor's mob," and the New York Doctors' Riot (as described in chapter one); many more followed across the country in areas near medical schools. Like Shippen Jr., John Collins Warren was attacked in his own home. In 1788 Charles F. Wiesenthal's anatomical school in Baltimore was mobbed, and the body of an executed murderer they were dissecting was taken.[42] After the body of a young woman was taken from her grave in Connecticut and ended up in Yale College in 1824, a mob raided the college for days, and destroyed property.[43] In 1830 Vermont's Castleton Medical College was the site of the "Hubbardton Raid," when 300 residents stormed the college looking for the body of a woman who was disinterred, which they found, headless.[44] The event was later turned into a song that retold the story of the raid, which featured the following lines:

> They pulled up a board from the floor,
> From this ancient seat of learning,
> And saw the body of the missing wife,
> The headless body of the exhumed woman,
> Thrust into a cramped up corner.
> These rustic raiders stood horrified
> Before this awful spectacle!
> This awful deed committed by the students
> In this ancient seat of learning,
> By the students of Castleton Medical College.
> The husband identified the remains,
> Could say they were his wife's, under oath,
> The body that was stolen from the graveyard.
> From the sacred graveyard in Hubbardton,
> From the land of battle, but not of song.[45]

Joseph Nash McDowell, known as "Mad Doctor McDowell" for his exploits, taught anatomy at Jefferson Medical College in its early years, and went on to establish the Missouri Medical College in St. Louis. McDowell kept a store of Revolutionary War-era weapons in the college that he had purchased from the government, and also obtained cannons, which he planned to use in a scheme to take land in Northern California (a harebrained plan that never came to fruition).[46] However, in 1849 he found a chance to use the weapons when he was suspected, falsely, of killing the wife of a wealthy German immigrant to dissect her. Three cannons were placed on the top floor of the building, ready for the oncoming mob of hundreds of people, McDowell leading his students in the fight, when the police intervened and defused the situation; the missing woman was later found alive and well in the company of another man.[47]

Physicians hired body snatchers to distance themselves from the unsavory crime of body snatching, offloading risk and paying for plausible deniability. Doctors couldn't stop riots, but they developed ingenious ways of concealing the dead in the event of one. Once, when a young woman died of a strange ailment, McDowell dug up her body with two of his students and took it to his college. Word got out, and McDowell was informed that people were coming to take her back, and he hid her body in the college's rafters. But before he could leave, men with guns were already in the college, and he claimed to have pretended to be a cadaver next to the other bodies; one of the men said as they passed him, partially covered in cloth, "Here is a fellow who died in his boots; I guess he is a fresh one."[48] He was also a spiritualist, and claimed he did this with the help of his dead mother, so it was not always clear what to believe in McDowell's tall tales.

According to Frederick C. Waite, medical colleges usually had places to hide cadavers; searches or riots were common enough that they were factored into how medical schools and dissecting rooms were built. Some colleges hid bodies in roof structures, such as a cupola, accessible only through a hidden trap door, where bodies were hoisted in by a system of pulleys.[49] Before a search of Columbian Medical College in D.C., the college's demonstrator of anatomy removed a part of the flooring and hid the body beneath it.[50] Once the search was complete, the body was taken out for dissection. Ohio's Homeopathic Medical College had a trap door in the floor where they kept bodies in a tank.[51]

In 1807 the building Dr. John B. Davidge used to teach anatomy in Baltimore was destroyed in an anatomy riot. Its successor, Davidge Hall, which is still in use today, was built with this experience in mind: the dissecting room on the second floor was made intentionally difficult to access, with a maze-like series of staircases and doors and hidden stairways and exits to escape in the event of a riot. Some medical schools had secret arrangements with the police, who notified them before searches were conducted so they had time to hide bodies in their prearranged hiding places.[52]

Medical schools also had to be wary of competing schools. A history of the Philadelphia Anatomical Rooms describes a time when "subjects unusually scarce, a fresh cadaver was stolen from this building at night and conveyed across the roof to the other [competing anatomy school]. Being too closely guarded for another Stygian journey back, and the offense not being indictable at law, even he [the Anatomical Rooms' janitor] was foiled."[53] The proprietors of the Philadelphia Anatomical Rooms were in a bind: they couldn't complain to the police that a body they had stolen was stolen from them, and so they were simply out of luck. At least one professor of anatomy, Dr. Moses Gunn, took bodies with him two separate times when he accepted new teaching positions in different states, much to the annoyance of the colleges he left behind, which could do nothing in response, given that they were not lawfully obtained in the first place.[54]

However, competing physicians could sometimes be accommodating:

> One night rival demonstrators met in a burying ground, out for the same body, and although strong personal friends they came nearly to shovel blows; when, however, the one proved his rights by priority of arrival, the other waived his claim to the stiff and assisted in the snatching. Another night, rivals scouted about a burying ground to get a body each had located during the funeral services earlier in the day; each party heard the other; each had visions of police officers and station houses, and they sneaked out of the grounds; but in about an hour they returned by different paths; the first arrival was given all the assistance that time would permit.[55]

Laws that prohibited body snatching were not very effective because they didn't address the root cause of body snatching: that there weren't enough bodies for dissection from legal sources. If one body snatcher was caught, another would take their place, and the trade would continue. The first law to address such supply issues dates back to 1540, when London's United Company of Barber Surgeons was given permission to dissect four executed criminals per year, which was later increased to six in 1663 by Charles II, "for their further and better knowledge, instruction, insight, learning, and experience in the said science or faculty of surgery."[56]

Judges sometimes added dissection as a posthumous punishment for felony convictions, but the 1752 Murder Act, an English law, mandated that executed murderers be dissected. The purpose of the law was to deter the crime of murder, but a byproduct of the law was that it provided doctors with a legal supply of bodies. The precedent this law set was followed in colonial America, including Pennsylvania. It even made its way into the first laws of New England, The Body of Liberties, used by the Massachusetts Bay Colony in 1641:

> No man condemned to dye shall be put to death within fower dayes next after his condemnation, unles the Court see spetiall cause to the contrary, or in case of martiall law, nor shall the body of any man so put to death be unburied 12 howers unlesse it be in case of Anatomie.[57]

Dissection wasn't used just to deter murder. In 1784 Massachusetts attempted to discourage the practice of dueling by requiring that anyone who died in a duel be dissected, or "secured and buried without a coffin, with a stake drove through the body at or near the usual place of execution…within ten miles of the town or place where the person was killed, otherwise the body shall in like manner be buried in the most public road in the town or place where the fact was committed."[58] Both were seen as equal punishments. If someone was executed for killing their opponent in a duel, they would be dissected after their death. Again, the supply of bodies for anatomists was a byproduct of the law, but there were too few to meet the needs of medical schools.

The first American law that supplied bodies explicitly for medical education was the same law that first prohibited body snatching in the country: New York's 1789 anatomy law. It was also the first to authorize dissection.[59] While dissection was never illegal, the law was silent on the matter. It was a gray area, which was why it was conducted quietly, as anatomists had to worry more about how the public would respond to their activities, such as with riots, than the law. In addition, New York's law codified the British precedent that judges could add dissection as an extra punishment for executed criminals, not just for felonies like murder, but also arson or burglary (which were removed as capital crimes in 1796).[60] Starting in 1790, the ability for judges to add dissection as punishment became federal law.[61] New Jersey passed a similar law in 1796.[62]

While New York's law was limited to the bodies of executed criminals, other states would expand who could be dissected. Connecticut's 1824 supply law added the unclaimed dead in the state's prison.[63] In 1831 Massachusetts passed a law after lobbying by the medical community that many consider to be the first true modern anatomy act because it made the unclaimed dead in *all* of the state's public institutions available for dissection; not just prisoners, but people who died in almshouses, hospitals, or other public institutions were eligible for dissection. This greatly increased the number of those eligible for dissection, and would be a key feature of future anatomy acts, including Pennsylvania's. Families or friends had 36 hours to claim bodies; otherwise, they were free to be dissected.

Massachusetts's law was, to say the least, controversial, as similar laws that followed would be, because dissection was historically a punishment for murder—reserved for only the worst of crimes—but with this law was now effectively a punishment for being poor. A key phrase in such laws, repeated verbatim from Massachusetts's law, was that it applied to the bodies of those "required to be buried at the public expense." The unclaimed included not just people who died in public institutions, primarily the almshouse, without families to claim and bury them, but families who couldn't afford to pay that expense. It also ignored the wishes of the people who died, as virtually none would have willingly donated their bodies for dissection. The law reflected an attitude that the involuntary donation of the bodies of the poor to science was the least they could do to pay back their debt to society, that the poor were to blame for their station in life, and could be treated like criminals. The term "unclaimed" made it sound like the law didn't target the poor, which obscured what was actually happening. It was a fact that physicians did their best to downplay, and many argued that such laws did not discriminate against the poor. John Collins Warren and other Massachusetts physicians wrote in a circular regarding the law:

> So far as the poor are concerned, it is for their especial benefit, that all physicians should be enabled to learn Anatomy thoroughly and practise [*sic*] it occasionally during life. Riches may procure medical or surgical skill, at whatever cost, and from any distance. And so long as the rich are willing to pay for this skill at its highest rate, a few individuals will be found, who will seek it abroad or at home, at immense expense, or personal sacrifice and risk. But the poor must be dependent for medical and surgical relief upon those who are nearest to them; and, generally, not upon those who have had the *most* opportunities of acquiring skill in the long-continued practice of their profession.[64]

Of course, the law benefitted the poor, as it did all by advancing medicine, but it still disproportionately affected them.

Connecticut and New Hampshire passed similar laws as those of Massachusetts but Connecticut repealed its laws just a year later, and New Hampshire eight years later.[65] They weren't exactly popular laws, with the public or most legislators. They were generally passed after lobbying from the medical community, and especially after a body-snatching scandal or riot increased public pressure for a legislative response to deal with a problem most, other than the medical community, would rather ignore. While today it seems obvious that dissection is necessary for the progress of medicine, and the benefits as a result of it, doctors were far ahead of the public in understanding the importance of the practice to the advance of medicine. Many simply didn't believe it was necessary, that doctors and medical students were motivated by a kind of morbid, blasphemous curiosity:

> The public at large looked upon body-snatching as contrary to all the established prejudices of humanity and did not care whether anatomy was studied or not, overlooking its paramount importance to the medical man. The profession, on the other hand, had a conscientious desire to know all about the body they were going to treat, which desire could easily be strained into an intention to obtain the knowledge in spite of the public. These two attitudes were utterly irreconcilable, and, as is the case when people see things from different standpoints, a good deal of bitter feeling was occasioned.[66]

Massachusetts's law also predated the United Kingdom's 1832 Anatomy Act by one year, which ended body snatching in Britain for good, also by appropriating the poor, but without the restrictions that limited the effectiveness of Massachusetts's law. The law consigned those who died in workhouses, prisons, and hospitals for medical education, unless they were claimed within 48 hours. It is often said that Burke and Hare's heinous crimes led to the passage of the Anatomy Act, but it was actually the London Burkers that finally spurred legislation.

The Bethnal Green Gang, as they were also known, turned from body snatching to burking and got caught in November 1831, when John Bishop and James May attempted to sell the unusually fresh body of a young Italian boy, an orphan, to King's College's anatomy school. When the demonstrator of anatomy examined the boy he purchased, he found "a wound on the head; the breast bone was injured, and all the teeth extracted, but the body appeared to have been in good health at the moment of death" (the teeth were extracted to sell them, a sideline of London's body snatchers).[67] The demonstrator contacted the authorities, and John Bishop, James May, Thomas Williams and Michael Shields were arrested for murder. Bishop and Williams confessed to multiple murders, and claimed that they drugged, then drowned and suffocated, their victims in a well. Bishop and Williams were executed and dissected, while May, who was not involved in the murders, was sentenced to "transportation" (to a penal colony), but died soon after. Shields was let free, as his only role in the crime was that he was hired to deliver the body. The possibility of "burking" would frequently be invoked by anatomists in support of future American anatomy laws, despite the fact that it, luckily, very rarely happened.

Unlike Britain's Anatomy Act, Massachusetts's failed to end body snatching in the state. The effectiveness of the law was limited by exceptions, which helped it get passed, such as that the law applied only to Boston, not the entire state, which limited the pool of available bodies. New York's supply law was further limited by the fact that it only applied to executed criminals. While the practice soon became nonexistent in Britain, America's patchwork, state-by-state approach kept body snatching alive and well in the country even into the 20th century. With no federal legislation, for body snatching to end, it had to be addressed nationally. Body snatchers sometimes disinterred the dead across state lines, which was less risky because the sheriff in the affected state only had jurisdiction to search there.[68]

New York and Massachusetts's supply laws were the only two in force and not repealed in the first half of the 19th century, but by 1850 all medical schools required anatomy education for graduation, and even more bodies were needed for dissection.[69] New York's 1854 "Bone Bill"—"An Act to Promote Medical Science and Protect Burial Grounds"—was modeled on Massachusetts's law, and had similar restrictions that limited its effectiveness.

Pennsylvania followed next. For the medical center of the country, dense with medical schools, it was odd that no law had been passed before; perhaps it wasn't needed, given that the almshouse was already a reliable source, and the city's potter's fields, and the secret agreements that facilitated the plunder of the city's dead. In 1863 the Pennsylvania legislature debated a bill called "An Act to Facilitate Anatomical Researches."[70] No riot had spurred consideration of a law, but a year before, Philadelphia's almshouse, then known as Old Blockley, had built a vault to prevent body snatching. While the vault failed to stop the practice, it may have led the state's medical community to lobby to protect their most important supply of bodies.

The bill legalized the transportation and receipt of unclaimed bodies for dissection in Pennsylvania medical schools. Transcripts of the debates provide a detailed look into arguments presented by both sides. The raging Civil War was a backdrop of the debate, and supporters of the law suggested that the act would better prepare doctors to treat soldiers. Opponents of the bill pointed out, correctly, that the devastation of the war provided plentiful opportunities for practice. However, physicians sought a long-term solution to the supply problem. The problem was framed as one that put physicians in an impossible situation: they could be held liable for malpractice, yet were not given sufficient means to gain the skill necessary to perform their job well. According to supporters of the law, physicians were *forced* to "pursue the horrible system to which they are now compelled to resort—to violate the graves of the dead in order to obtain the necessary subjects for anatomical research."[71]

More fundamental issues were also at play. Supporters of the bill called for a focus on reason and judgment, rather than feelings and sentimentality, in considering the bill. By "sentimentality," supporters seemed to mean the belief in the need to care for the body after death: "I imagine that if either the gentleman from Warren or the gentleman from Lancaster, were so unfortunate as to have a broken leg, he would be glad to have something else than sentiment to cure it."[72] One opponent of the law expressed the view, "the great Author of our being has implanted this feeling within us, and I doubt not for some wise purpose. We see this feeling manifested in the care bestowed by the people of all nations upon the resting places of the dead…It is a feeling universal."[73] In other words, even the poor, and the unclaimed poor, deserved a proper burial. One body snatcher in 1875 echoed the physicians' arguments in their defense: "A Philadelphia body-snatcher defends his business on the ground that the dead are clay, and so long as the spirit is in Heaven it matters not what becomes of the mortal shell."[74]

A supporter expressed the opposite view:

> We owe a higher duty to the living than to the dead—that when it has pleased the Almighty to cut off our pilgrimage on earth, it is a matter of minor consequence what becomes of the poor shell that once contained an immortal soul—that if we have prepared our immortal part so that it is ready for heaven, it matters but little whether our bodies rot in the earth, are devoured by wild beasts, are lost in the ocean, or whether they contribute some benefit to those who survive us. I would say, let my body contribute to the benefit of those who survive me rather than be nothing but an offence to them.[75]

In reality, most doctors, like the general public, with some exceptions, avoided being dissected themselves at all costs. When Mr. Shannon noted that "burial is a Christian duty," Mr. Trimmer responded, "Is it not a Christian duty to take care of them also while they are sick?"[76] At one point another opponent of the legislation said, "notwithstanding the frosts upon my head, I have the sympathies of the human heart, which I am very sorry that he does not possess."[77] Opponents of the bill noted their support for the progress of medicine, but never offered a solution to the problem. They simply denied that it was a problem, that there were already enough bodies to go around for medical education.

But the solution proposed targeted the poor, which opponents of the bill recognized:

> The institutions of the State of Pennsylvania are founded upon the principle of the entire equality of all men before the law; yet this bill, because a man is poor and friendless, proposes that his body shall be handed over for the purpose of

> mutilation. I esteem as highly as any one the importance, for the sake of medical science and anatomical and surgical researches, of having these dissections; but, sir, I would not sanction them by any public act of the Legislature.[78]
>
> I deny that we have any right to treat the poor with this sort of inhumanity. The poor are those who ought to be specially under the protection of the Commonwealth. The rich can take care of themselves.[79]

One speaker mockingly quoted the English poet Thomas Noel: "Rattle his bones over the stones! He is only a pauper whom nobody owns!"[80]

Supporters of the law argued that the poor would benefit most from the law, and that the feelings of family or friends of the deceased would not be injured because they could claim them, but this ignored the fact that many if not most could not afford to claim those who died in the almshouse. The need for bodies, and the medical benefits of dissection, did not change the cultural understanding of dissection as punishment, a punishment anatomists were attempting to reserve primarily for those who resided in the almshouse. The bill failed to pass due to lack of support.

A new version of the bill was written by Dr. William S. Forbes in 1867. Forbes sought the help of the College of Physicians of Philadelphia, the oldest private medical society in the country, to present to the legislature a new law to address body snatching, which they assented to. While it initially failed to pass, the college enlisted the help of Wilmer Worthington, senator and doctor, to push for reconsideration of the bill, which was again rebuffed, but his efforts helped enable a committee that included Forbes to go before the legislature to defend the bill.[81] The arguments for and against the bill were similar—that doctors did not have the bodies they needed to become skilled surgeons, but were liable for malpractice, and the possibility of burking. But this time, the law was passed. While most legislators shared widespread beliefs regarding care for the dead, and thought that denying paupers this right was unjust, most also accepted that anatomists required bodies to advance medical science and treatment. Faced with this dilemma, and the lobbying of the increasingly influential Philadelphia medical community, the law was passed.

Officially known as an act "For the Promotion of Medical Science, and to prevent the Traffic in Human Bodies in the City of Philadelphia and County of Allegheny," unofficially as the "Ghastly Act," the law read:

> SECTION 1. Be it enacted by the Senate and House of Representatives of the Commonwealth of Pennsylvania, in General Assembly met, and it is hereby enacted by the authority of the same, That any public officer in the City of Philadelphia or County of Allegheny, having charge thereof or control over the same, shall give permission to any physician or surgeon of the same city or county, upon his request made therefor, to take the bodies of deceased persons required to be buried at the public expense, to be by him used within the State for the advancement of medical science, preference being given to medical schools, public and private; and said bodies to be distributed to and among the same, equitably, the number assigned to each being proportioned to that of its students; provided, however, that if the deceased person, during his or her last sickness, of his or her own accord, shall request to be buried; or if any person, claiming to be, and satisfying the proper authorities that he or she is of kindred to the deceased, shall ask to have the body for burial, it shall be surrendered for interment; or, if such deceased person was a stranger or traveler, who died suddenly, the body shall be buried, and shall not be handed over as aforesaid.
>
> SECTION 2. Every physician or surgeon, before receiving any such dead body, shall give to the proper authorities surrendering the same to him, a sufficient bond that each body shall be used only for the promotion of medical science within this State; and whosoever shall use such body or bodies for any other purpose, or shall remove the same beyond the limits of this State; and whosoever shall sell or buy such body or bodies for any other purpose, or shall remove the same beyond the limits of this State; and whosoever shall sell or buy such body or bodies, or in any way traffic in the same, shall be deemed guilty of a misdemeanor, and shall, on conviction, be imprisoned for a term not exceeding five years, at hard labor, in the county jail.[82]

Note the change in the name of the act; stopping body snatching now had equal billing with the advancement of science. The law effectively legalized a long-standing practice: taking the bodies of the poor from the Philadelphia almshouse against their will for dissection. The law did note that if "the deceased person, during his or her last sickness, of his or her own accord, shall request to be buried…it shall be surrendered for interment," but it is unclear exactly what this meant in practice. If inmates were required to pay for their burial, this was highly unlikely to happen. If it was free of charge, whether inmates were informed of this option or if it was ever invoked is an open question. Even before the passage of the law, the almshouse allowed the dissection of the "unclaimed" dead, and made no mention of inmates claiming themselves. Regardless, if the almshouse did bury inmates who requested it, they didn't stay in the graveyard for long given the rampant body snatching in the institution.

One factor that led to the bill's success was a significant concession: it was limited in geographic scope to Philadelphia and Allegheny County (Pittsburgh); the latter was included at the request of a legislator who represented the area. Philadelphia, dense with medical schools, would be able to obtain the city's unclaimed dead, chiefly from the almshouse, but also the dead of other public institutions, such as the prison. The Philadelphia Anatomical Association, composed of anatomists from the different schools, public and private, distributed bodies based on the size of classes.

But the law had another limitation: it was not mandatory. People in charge of the dead in public institutions, according to the law, "shall give permission" for anatomists to have bodies, but it was not required. The law lacked an enforcement mechanism, and so Philadelphia anatomists' supply could be cut off any time, ensuring that supply issues, and body snatching, would continue. Despite this, the public was falsely reassured by the passage of the law that it had ended body snatching, but it continued in areas the law covered—Philadelphia, Allegheny County—and in areas it didn't.

In 1869, two years after the law passed, a medical student stole the body of an executed murderer buried in Butler, Pennsylvania's woods because no cemetery would take his body, and took it to Allegheny.[83] In 1873 the body of Thomas Munco, a wealthy farmer from Washington County, Pennsylvania, was found drowned in the Schuylkill River.[84] At the time of discovery, the identity of the individual was not known, and the body was taken to the coroner. On the way there, the driver of the coroner's wagon pawned the watch that was found on the body. The body ended up at the University of Pennsylvania, much to the consternation of the missing man's family. If the identity of a person was unknown, the person was supposed to be buried, according to the law.

In 1875 the superintendent of the City Burial Grounds, William Taylor, was charged with body snatching, selling bodies that were supposed to be buried there to medical schools.[85] The charges were eventually dropped, but further controversy erupted the next year, when the sister of a man from Baltimore, who had recently moved to Philadelphia after her brother was buried there, came to the city to rebury him in another cemetery, but his body couldn't be found.[86] A Philadelphia newspaper noted in 1876 that bodies were taken from the City Burial Ground "almost daily," bodies that shouldn't have been eligible for dissection.[87] It also noted that "Neighbors to the Potter's Field say that the sight of a grave being dug there is a rare one."[88]

Before Pennsylvania prohibited body snatching in 1849 and passed an anatomy law in 1867, body snatching had flourished in the state, especially in Philadelphia, for the better part of a century. Originally, laws that provided bodies for dissection were a form of punishment. As awareness of body snatching increased with the opening of medical schools around America, laws were passed in a piecemeal fashion, state by state, to punish body snatchers, and physicians like McKnight or professional body snatchers stole bodies, primarily from Black cemeteries or public institutions like Philadelphia's almshouse. But simply punishing body snatchers wasn't enough given how lucrative the trade was, and how infrequently the penalties were enforced. Eventually states started to address the causes of body snatching, starting in New York, with the gradual expansion of the bodies available for dissection, culminating in allowing the bodies of all unclaimed dead who died in public institutions for dissection in Massachusetts—and soon after, in the United Kingdom—and in 1867, Pennsylvania.

With the limitations of Pennsylvania's 1867 law, controversies continued until 1882, when the most infamous case of body snatching in Philadelphia and Pennsylvania history put body snatching, and the limitations of the law, in the spotlight. Three body snatchers were arrested for stealing bodies from a Black cemetery in Philadelphia to supply Jefferson Medical College, and the college's demonstrator of anatomy, William S. Forbes, would face a high-profile trial for, ironically, violating a law that he wrote. It would also lead to a revised Pennsylvania anatomy law, one that the convicted body-snatcher-turned-state-senator William J. McKnight played a key role in passing. The revised law would end body snatching in the state for good, and become a model followed by other states, by strengthening the law and mandating the appropriation of the bodies of the poor.

CHAPTER 7

"Jefferson's Resurrection Keys"

Body Snatching on Trial

> In cases of this kind, where the necessities of society are in conflict with the law, and with public opinion, the crime consists...not in the deed, but in permitting its discovery.
>
> —EDWARD WARREN, 1874[1]

Louis N. Megargee, city editor of *The Philadelphia Press*, was on a stakeout. He had been staring at the same stable for three weeks when, finally, a wagon departed at a suspiciously late hour on December 4, 1882. During the day the wagon's driver, Frank McNamee, delivered mail for the United States Post Office Department, but Megargee knew that at night he conveyed a very different kind of cargo. Two carriages containing six men tailed McNamee: five reporters from *The Press* and a Pinkerton, or private detective, named William Henderson. They stopped near the intersection of Passyunk Avenue and Broad Street in South Philadelphia and made the rest of their journey on foot. They knew exactly where McNamee was headed.

Lebanon Cemetery was established on what was then Philadelphia's outskirts in 1849 by Jacob Clement White Sr., an entrepreneur and one of the city's most affluent residents. It was the first of two nonsectarian Black "rural" cemeteries to open in Philadelphia that year—Olive Cemetery followed shortly after—a place where Philadelphia's Black community could bury their dead with dignity.[2] Barred from white cemeteries, Black Philadelphians had few choices of where they could bury their dead, an issue that reached the Supreme Court of Pennsylvania in 1876.

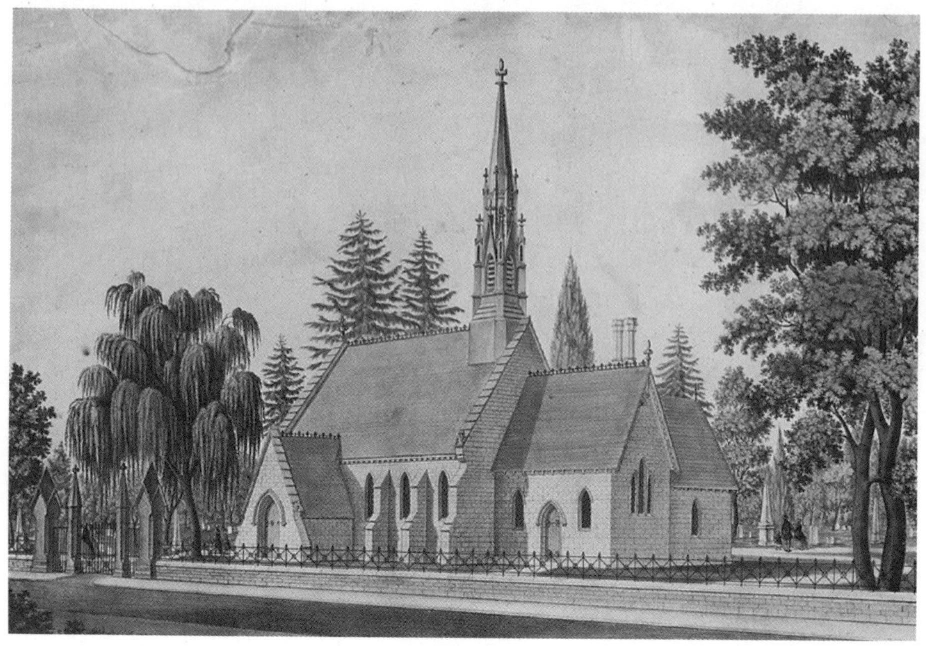

The Chapel of Lebanon Cemetery, 1850. (Wikimedia Commons)

Henry Jones, a formerly enslaved man who became a successful caterer, wished to be buried in Mount Moriah Cemetery. Henry and his wife Margaret purchased a portion of a lot from a white lot holder named William H. Boileau, where Margaret's sister was buried without controversy.[3] After Henry passed, Margaret was informed just 15 minutes before his funeral that her request to bury him in Moriah was denied by the cemetery association:

> So great is the opposition on the part of a large majority of our many thousand lot-holders to the interment of colored persons in the cemetery among their deceased friends and relatives, that, if we were to permit it, it would probably lead to acts of violence and breaches of the peace, large numbers of the dead already interred therein would be removed, as has been expressly threatened in many instances, the association would be financially ruined and compelled to leave the thousands of existing graves to the result of abandonment and neglect.[4]

The Supreme Court was not convinced, and deemed the association's actions "arbitrary and unreasonable" and decided in Margaret's favor.[5] But she feared for the safety of her husband's grave and expressed her intention to bury him in Lebanon Cemetery instead, although he may have actually been buried in St. James the Less Episcopal Church.[6]

Many prominent Black Philadelphians were buried in Lebanon, such as Octavius Catto, an educator, civil rights activist, and baseball player, as well as veterans of the Civil War, like Captain A. Oscar Jones, and members of the United States Colored Troops (USCT). Jacob Clement White Jr., the son of the cemetery's founder and secretary of the cemetery's association, later told a reporter, "People have asked me if I thought the dead were perfectly safe so far away from the settled part of the city, but I have always said that I believed there was no danger."[7] Philadelphia-area rural cemeteries like Laurel Hill, and likely Mount Moriah as well, had protections for its dead—gates, walls, receiving vaults, watchmen, dogs let loose to act as sentinels—not just for potential body snatchers, but grave robbers, people intent on the theft of grave goods or the ransom of bodies of the wealthy people interred there. In a story about graveyard precautions in cemeteries like Laurel Hill, a Pennsylvania newspaper reported that except for the purposes of medical education, "Nobody wants to steal the flesh and bones of poor people"; unless someone who was wealthy died of an unusual ailment, their body was usually stolen for non-medical reasons, which was what the protections were for.[8] But Lebanon had few protections, and its superintendent who lived in the cemetery's chapel was in the pay of body snatchers.

McNamee drew his wagon to a halt in front of Lebanon Cemetery and waited while his two passengers, "Dutch" Pillet and Levi Chew, entered a gap in the fence. A horrifying sight awaited the pair on the consecrated ground: six dead bodies. But they were not surprised. The superintendent and grave digger, Levi's brother Robert Chew, left them the "small-pox cases" (the code word for bodies)—for three dollars apiece. When Robert couldn't get away with burying empty coffins, he marked recently dug graves, the freshest, and Pillet and Levi exhumed them:

> If business was brisk and time precious only one half of the grave—the portion toward the head—was dug anew. Then the head of the coffin was broken, a rope tied around the neck of the corpse and the body pulled out by main force. It was quickly stripped of every article of clothing and these cast in the grave, none of them ever being retained through a fear that its possession by a living person might lead to detection.[9]

Dutch and Levi loaded the six corpses into the wagon and departed for Jefferson Medical College. Founded in 1824, Jefferson was the city's second medical school after the University of Pennsylvania, where illustrious anatomists like Samuel D. Gross and Thomas Dent Mütter (whose collection forms the basis of today's Mütter Museum) taught, and rivaled Penn in national stature (today the school is known as the Sidney Kimmel Medical College, part of Thomas Jefferson University, which merged with Philadelphia University in 2017).[10] To the body snatchers that night was a business transaction, one they had done many times before. To Megargee it was one of the biggest scoops of his career. Not content to just report the story, Megargee and *The Press* became an integral part of it.

The first hints of a body-snatching ring were dropped by joking Jefferson medical students. After a bartender known as Jim at Dooner's restaurant on Chestnut Street died, a medical student who talked with the owner quipped that he had seen Jim after he had been buried in Lebanon. The owner told a reporter what he heard, and *The Press*'s investigation began. The scope of the plot they uncovered was staggering. Lebanon Cemetery had been plundered for at least 20 years: "It is no exaggeration to state that the bodies that have been stolen far outnumber those that have been permitted to remain."[11] The origins of the arrangement are murky. There was an "old man, now dead…[who] went the way—or at least a part of the way—of his stock in trade"; the transportation of the bodies was managed by a "public carter, whose stand for years was at Tenth and Market streets."[12] Robert's brother Solomon Butcher was also said to have supplied bodies for Jefferson from the cemetery.

John Mayer, a German immigrant and saloonkeeper, got into the business when one of his patrons, a doctor from Jefferson who shipped bodies from Maryland to Philadelphia, came up short in his supply. Mayer approached and struck a deal with Robert to supply the college: "They bury five blacks a day there, sometimes, and nobody thinks anything of 'em. Why should they? They never were any good," he told a reporter.[13] After a pay dispute with Jefferson, McNamee took over Mayer's operation. *The Press* discovered the resurrection ring in the spring of 1882, but the body snatchers ceased their operation in the summer. Classes weren't in session in the summer because the heat putrefied bodies too quickly, and were instead held in the colder months so they lasted longer. Megargee was determined to catch the body snatchers in the act when they resumed their work in the winter.

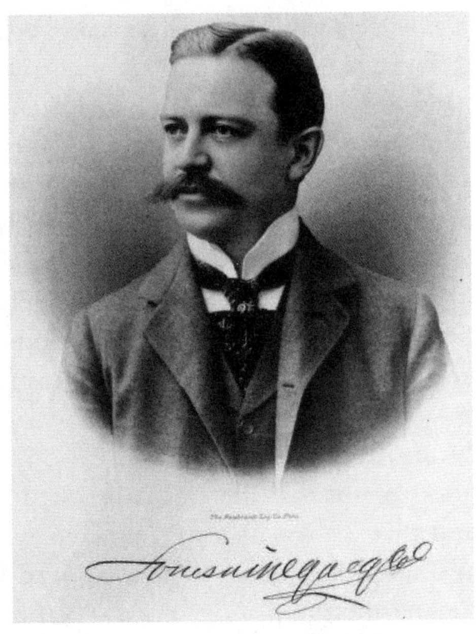

Portrait of Louis N. Megargee, who uncovered a body-snatching ring between Lebanon Cemetery and Jefferson Medical College. (Internet Archive)

The five reporters and Pinkerton waited on opposite sides of the road as a wagon approached. Normally it wouldn't be hard to confirm that it was McNamee's: his name and business address were emblazoned on its sides, a sign of incaution, or an attempt to use his legitimate business as a way to disguise his illegitimate one. But little could be made out in the darkness. Originally their plan was to stretch out a rope across the road closer to the cemetery to surprise them, but they ran out of time. Instead, one of *The Press* men stepped into the road and yelled, "Hold on! I want to see you."[14] He recognized Levi, pulled out his revolver, and yelled, "Drop those lines! Hold up your hands. Quick, or I will blow a hole through you."[15] The other men followed suit, and six guns were aimed squarely at the three body snatchers.

McNamee, Dutch, and Levi were arrested and taken to the local Pinkerton Detective Agency. Megargee had a warrant for McNamee and the others' arrest based on his testimony, for the charge of "conspiracy to commit a misdemeanor," approved by a magistrate, who deputized him as a constable to carry it out.[16] According to an 1873 Philadelphia law, cemetery employees could arrest and transport violators of cemetery laws for prosecution after taking an oath before a magistrate, and apparently journalists as well, if they made a convincing enough case.[17]

The Press and Pinkerton later returned to the cemetery and arrested Robert. Andrew "Yank" Mullen who worked for McNamee was also named on the warrant, but was not involved in the body snatching that night. Mullen appeared at McNamee's stable the next day and was taken to the Pinkerton agency, but McNamee pleaded for Mullen to be able to deliver mail as part of his legitimate business, and they let him go. Perhaps not surprisingly, he went missing, and did not appear in court at the appointed time. A key piece of evidence was found on McNamee: keys to Jefferson Medical College, which implicated the college. McNamee claimed he was just the driver and was asked to haul the bodies and given the keys by a stranger. The six stolen bodies were taken to Eberle's stable on Sansom Street, below 9th; the owner later complained that the journalists lied to him about the wagon's contents, and that he was accosted by a crowd of people looking for the bodies, and intended to sue for damages to his business.[18]

The next day's edition of *The Philadelphia Press* exposed what would become the city's most infamous case of body snatching, in a multi-page story that featured sensational headlines like "Graveyard Ghouls Arrested with a Cargo of Corpses," "The Ghastly Work Done for Jefferson Medical College," and "LEBANON CEMETERY ALMOST EMPTY."[19] Its content was equally sensational, and probably embellished for dramatic effect. *The Press* claimed that its reporters observed the body snatchers at Lebanon and Jefferson before they made their arrest—that two of the journalists pretended to be drunk on the road near the cemetery to avoid detection, and posed as medical students to gather information.

In reality, body snatching at Lebanon Cemetery was an open secret. An anonymous source, the saloonkeeper John Mayer, talked to the press in 1880 about how he stole bodies from Lebanon, but not where they were delivered: "Well, the old Lebanon cemetery, on the Passyunk road used to be our cheese. We 'ad the sexton of the place all right and got enough 'stiffs' from that place to supply the doctors."[20] While only mentioned in passing in a Pennsylvania newspaper, it was there for anyone to see, but seemed to have no impact. Most may have believed body snatching was a thing of the past with the state's 1867 anatomy law, notwithstanding the scandals around the coroner's office and potter's field and after its passage.

Philadelphia's detectives only investigated crimes that people reported; evidently a complaint was never made to them.[21] Some have suggested it may not have been a crime the police felt inclined to investigate, especially since its victims were African Americans.[22] Just the year before the mayor of Philadelphia appointed four Black officers to the force, after which a number of officers quit in protest.[23] Megargee had recently exposed corruption in the Philadelphia Police Department, which might have affected his level of trust with the department, but in a later retelling of these events he wrote why he bypassed the police:

> While the object of the investigation was certainly praiseworthy, the journal conducting it, naturally, did not wish any rival to share in the result of its labors. Consequently it would not do to take police officials into the secret, the inevitable result of which would have been their mounting the house-tops and proclaiming to the city their vigilance and acumen. In order, therefore, to have authority for the arrest of the criminals, a warrant was secured from a magistrate whose secrecy could be absolutely relied upon.[24]

The Press were "muckrakers," journalists that exposed misdeeds in the pursuit of reform and, of course, to sell papers. Many points of the story seemed like self-advertisement for *The Press*: "the arrest, unprecedented in the history of newspaper enterprise, may hereafter confine students' scalpels to bodies given to science by the law."[25] Later issues devoted space to recounting the praise of other newspapers for their zeal in combating body snatching. Despite *The Press*'s sensationalism, or because of it, the story spread like wildfire to an outraged public, but the basic facts of the case were not in dispute.

The theft of bodies from a Black cemetery for an all-white medical school galvanized the Black Philadelphia community. The crime added insult to injury: Black Philadelphians were excluded from white cemeteries, yet targeted by body snatchers. That morning the six stolen bodies were taken to the morgue, where families and friends who had recently buried their loved ones in Lebanon filed in to identify the bodies, along with curious onlookers. According to *The Press*:

> When they were first admitted into the room where perhaps lay a brother, a sister, husband, mother or wife, their faces became almost livid with fear...tears streamed from their eyes as they recognized a friend or relative and occasionally the tear was dried and the eye flashed forth a look of anger and defiance as they heaped maledictions on the head of the rude disturbers of their sacred dead.[26]

The bodies were later reburied in Lebanon Cemetery.

That same day Black Philadelphians held an "indignation meeting" which, according to historian Michael E. Woods, was a forum for citizens to channel their anger into political action. The crowd's anger was directed at the body snatchers, Robert, and the cemetery's trustees, and while there were some outbursts in the audience that called for violence, before and after the meeting, it never materialized. The participants resolved to open graves in Lebanon Cemetery to determine how many bodies had been stolen.[27] Permits were obtained from the Health Office to exhume bodies, and when the graves were opened later that day the worst fears of many were confirmed: "Mothers wept over the graves of their babes," and "Fathers and brothers stood in little groupes [*sic*], and with set features and flashing eyes, swore by Almighty God to visit summary vengeance on the ghouls who had robbed them of their dead."[28]

In the days after, people continued to flood the cemetery, and the Health Office eventually stopped granting permits to open graves out of fear that the diseases people died of might spread. A second indignation meeting was held two days later where, by one count, over 600 people gathered.[29] The location of the meeting, Liberty Hall, was significant: the building was established in 1867 by and for African Americans.[30] The speakers overwhelmingly advocated for using the law to punish the body snatchers, although the same tension in the last meeting was still there, evident from the verbal outbursts of some in the audience—anger directed not just at the body snatchers but Lebanon's trustees, who had placed their trust in Robert.[31] The preamble and resolution of the indignation meeting was:

> We, citizens of Philadelphia, feeling the great outrage that has been perpetrated against us by the disgraceful robbery of graves in Lebanon Cemetery by a class of human fiends, whose names will always be looked upon as infamous, do protest against this outrage upon us as a people. Resolved, That our heartfelt and sincere thanks are hereby tendered to the proprietor of THE PRESS, to Mr. Louis N. Megargee and all those who were connected with making the arrests.[32]

In *The Press*, readers were greeted with a sensationalized crime and a heroic story of intrepid journalists enforcing the law. *The Press* and other white papers also played up the threat of Black violence, and spent far less time covering the ultimately peaceful, if fraught, indignation meetings of the Black community. The event was framed very differently in *The Christian Recorder*, one of the most influential Black newspapers of the 19th century. The Black community's response to the crime was organized and political, focused on using the law to punish the perpetrators, finding a long-term solution to the problem of body snatching, and self-reflection:

> It is to be hoped that the law authorities will search the whole affair to its very depths and allow none who in any way profited by the sacrilege to escape; Not a little of the responsibility rests upon the colored people themselves, owing to the wretched condition in which they allow the graves...to remain. When we as a class shall show the respect for our dead that others show, such outrages will measurably cease.[33]

Lebanon's problems stemmed in part from mismanagement by Robert, who left the cemetery he was entrusted with in a state of disrepair, according to *The Philadelphia Inquirer*:

> The burial grounds are in a very dilapidated condition, and showed a want of care on the part of those having charge of its superintendence. Only a few of the lots are inclosed [*sic*] by railings, and the tombstones in many instances have fallen or been thrown out of position. Some of the graves showed evidence of having been tampered with, from the appearance of having been recently dug, although no interments have taken place in the same spot for a long time. In other places the tops of the graves had sunken beneath the surface. This state of affairs was noticeable along the eastern side of the cemetery, where bodies have been lately buried. A boy who was walking along there yesterday struck something hard with a stick, which, upon investigation, proved to be a human skull. A crowd of curious colored people immediately collected, and in a few minutes other portions of the human skeleton were unearthed…It was explained by one of the bystanders who was familiar with the management of the cemetery, that this was the work of Robert Chew, the superintendent. It was the latter's practice, it is said, to have a grave dug in another part of the ground, and then as soon as the relatives and funeral mourners left the place to shift the body to the eastern part of the cemetery, whence it would be removed by McNamee and his colleagues to the dissecting room. This was called "shifting the bodies."[34]

Another story spurred by *The Press*'s activist journalism that focused on a Black cemetery in Harrisburg, Pennsylvania, shared similar problems that Lebanon had. *The Harrisburg Daily* ran a story with the sensational headline "GRAVES UNEARTHED IN A COLORED CEMETERY

BY DOGS," and painted a picture of a rundown cemetery (the Harris Free Cemetery) where dogs feasted on shallowly buried corpses.[35] The story described how the cemetery lacked funding, how individuals lacked funds to pay for burials (which resulted in improper burials), and how the sexton refused to work due to lack of pay. The cemetery also experienced a white-led race riot five years previously which had caused significant damage. One newspaper argued that what happened in Lebanon Cemetery was beneficial for it: "it appeared that a number of bodies of colored persons had been taken from Lebanon Cemetery from trenches or deep pits in which dozens of dead bodies were buried in common, and which but for the regular relief would soon have been overflowing."[36] In reality, the bodies were dug that way intentionally by the superintendent to make them easier to steal, not out of negligence.[37]

The prisoners' first hearing the day after their arrest was thronged with people, many of them Black Philadelphians, some looking to get a glimpse of the ghouls, others to administer vigilante justice with the weapons they carried if they could only get their hands on them. The ringleader McNamee was a "short, well-built, bearded man" who previously served two years in prison for selling stolen goods, the "present manager of the Philadelphia and Atlantic express, proprietor of the Bryn Mawr baggage express, a public carter, a dealer in rags…a minor Republican politician of the Eighth ward," and a janitor.[38] Body snatching was just another side business. Dutch was a "rough looking specimen of the degraded outcast," blind in one eye, who worked for McNamee's legitimate mail delivery business.[39] Levi Chew worked for an undertaker. Robert was of course Lebanon Cemetery's superintendent, who claimed he didn't participate in body snatching because he was afraid of ghosts, a strange defense for someone who lived in a graveyard. Levi and his brother Robert were Black, while the other perpetrators were white.

The body snatchers, Megargee, and other witnesses were questioned to establish the facts of the case. Megargee testified that the keys found on McNamee fit Jefferson's locks. No lawyer would represent the body snatchers, and no one made bail, which was set at 5,000 dollars. After the hearing, the prisoners were herded to jail despite the large crowd gathered. Getting the prisoners from the office to the jail despite crowds was difficult, and they had to wait for the commotion to die down.

The next day's issue of *The Press* prominently displayed on its front page a facsimile of the keys that were found on McNamee, with the headline "Jefferson's Resurrection Keys. The Means by Which the Body-Snatchers Gained Entrance to the College."[40] The message was clear: Jefferson, or more specifically, its demonstrator of anatomy, William S. Forbes, was responsible for the crime, not just the body snatchers. Originally from Virginia, Forbes moved to Philadelphia to study at Jefferson. After graduating he had a long and varied career, as a resident physician in Pennsylvania Hospital, a volunteer surgeon in the British Army in the Crimean War, an instructor in his own private anatomy school in Philadelphia, a surgeon in the Civil War, and Jefferson's demonstrator in 1879. Like other demonstrators, it was his job to supply bodies for dissection, and when asked about the crime, college officials put the blame squarely on Forbes. If there was anyone who could follow Pennsylvania's 1867 anatomy law to the letter it was Forbes: after all, he wrote it. But Forbes also understood the reality that the law didn't provide enough bodies for anatomical education in the city, and that other, less savory sources were needed to meet such shortfalls.

At his first lecture after the revelations Forbes had trouble controlling his unruly students: "Gentleman…you are about to enter a noble career," Forbes said.[41] One student quipped, "Doubt it!"[42] The reaction of Jefferson students to the news of where Jefferson's bodies were supplied from was, to say the least, insensitive. After hearing about the indignation meeting, a student asked "'Are we to be mobbed?'…'I don't know,' answered the student addressed, 'but I shouldn't mind if we were. There are 600 of us [enrolled in the college], and I guess we might have some fun. We might make a few fresh stiffs too.'"[43] Students sang racist songs. They also threatened the college's Black janitor: "Jim, Dr. Forbes says you better keep your mouth shut. You are talking too much."[44] Police were stationed as guards at Jefferson and Lebanon Cemetery.

The general public was also horrified by the crime. Newspaper articles circulated about the defenses in white cemeteries to assure a fearful public, with headlines like "Guarding the Graves. A Timely

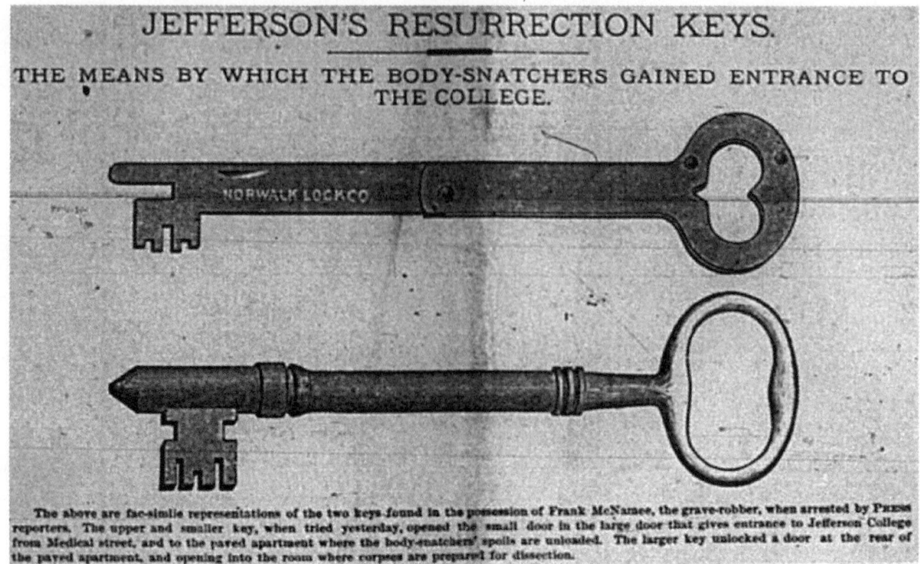

JEFFERSON'S RESURRECTION KEYS.

THE MEANS BY WHICH THE BODY-SNATCHERS GAINED ENTRANCE TO THE COLLEGE.

The above are fac-simile representations of the two keys found in the possession of Frank McNamee, the grave-robber, when arrested by PRESS reporters. The upper and smaller key, when tried yesterday, opened the small door in the large door that gives entrance to Jefferson College from Medical street, and to the paved apartment where the body-snatchers' spoils are unloaded. The larger key unlocked a door at the rear of the paved apartment, and opening into the room where corpses are prepared for dissection.

The keys to Jefferson found on body-snatcher Frank McNamee, which are in Thomas Jefferson University Archives today. (Author scan)

Suggestion For Our Cemetery Authorities. How the Allegheny and Uniondale Burial Grounds are Protected by Armed Patrols at Night—Breech-Loading Shot-Guns Ready for Instant Use."[45] Historian Alan C. Braddock pointed out that an advertisement in *The Press* that appeared soon after the crime, for a blackface minstrel show called "A Night in a Medical College," which addressed recent events, that drew large audiences.

At a second hearing a few days later, Forbes testified that he gave the keys to McNamee because he delivered legitimate bodies, and that he had no reason to believe they came from an illegitimate source. He claimed to have a policy of not asking questions, and that he didn't personally receive the bodies; his assistant did. Forbes said he paid McNamee five dollars for the hauling of bodies to the college, but sometimes more, which depended on the distance the bodies were hauled. When asked how Forbes knew what to pay McNamee if he didn't ask questions, he replied that McNamee told him if it came from a farther distance, such as the prison, and that he trusted him to tell the truth. When asked why he wasn't suspicious when McNamee brought six bodies of people who supposedly died in the prison on the same day, Forbes didn't have a convincing response. Generally, bodies from the prison were few and far between, and most came from the almshouse.

The trial of the four body snatchers followed not long after that month, and each were charged with six counts of violation of sepulchre. McNamee and Pillet initially pled not guilty, but, reportedly, once they discovered that the foreman of the jury was Black, they changed their pleas to guilty, because they believed they had no chance in a trial. The Chews pled not guilty and decided to let the jury decide their fate. When deliberations began, they were found guilty in less than a minute. When the foreman announced the verdict, he said, "Is there no law to hang them?"[46] In a stunning turn of events, during the trial Forbes was arrested and brought to court. Just as the body snatchers, he was held on 5,000 dollars bail.

McNamee was allowed to make a statement, and said that he had an explicit arrangement with Forbes to supply him with bodies from Lebanon Cemetery. McNamee told the court that he was initially hired by one of Forbes's assistants to haul a body from the county prison to Jefferson. He did this multiple times, and then was asked to haul bodies from Lebanon Cemetery, where the bodies were waiting for him to pick up. He hauled more bodies from Lebanon but claimed he wasn't paid, so he spoke to Forbes directly instead of his assistant. According to McNamee, it was then that they made the arrangement.

McNamee explained how the operation worked: Levi told McNamee bodies were ready, McNamee went to Forbes's house, and he handed him the keys. Once the job was done, someone would be waiting at night when he made the delivery with his assistants, and he was paid the next day, and would return the keys. McNamee claimed that Forbes told him he was doing nothing illegal: "No, the worst they can do is to discharge the men down at the burying ground; you do nothing but haul…I and some other gentleman went to Harrisburg and had a law passed making it criminal to take bodies out of the city or state…Do you think we would allow you to do wrong [?]"

Forbes made bail and was indicted, but his trial was postponed after the death of his father-in-law and the illness of another family member. Clearly, Forbes was given a degree of flexibility by virtue of his social standing. It's hard to imagine the same courtesy being paid to someone like McNamee, whose sentencing, along with the other body snatchers, was delayed until after Forbes's trial, which didn't resume for three months.

Before Forbes's trial there was movement on a revised anatomy law that would end body snatching for good in Philadelphia and Pennsylvania. While it was Forbes who wrote the 1867 law, it was William J. McKnight, a convicted body snatcher turned Pennsylvania state senator, who played a key role in pushing for a revised anatomy law for the state.[47] Since his conviction in 1857, McKnight had served as a surgeon in the Civil War, continued his private practice after, and became a state senator in 1880. At the time of the crime, he was also a student at Jefferson. McKnight was in a unique position, someone with direct experience of body snatching, ties to Jefferson's faculty, and political ties as a senator—all of which would prove critical in the passage of a revised anatomy law.[48]

As McKnight told it, he dined with William H. Pancoast, Jefferson's professor of anatomy (the head of Forbes's department) soon after the scandal broke, who wondered how the crime would impact the college. McKnight proposed that now was the time to secure changes to the existing anatomy law to make it more effective, and Pancoast questioned whether in the middle of the controversy was the right time to pursue change. McKnight said:

> The people of the city and State are excited, alarmed, and angered, and I would frame the "act to prevent the traffic in human bodies and to prevent the desecration of graveyards." This would appeal to the good sense of the people, as an effort, at least, in the right direction.[49]

In other words, McKnight wanted to frame the argument for the law as a means to end body snatching for good, which was exactly what the public wanted. He wasn't wrong, as the most drastic legal change usually happened after scandals like the one Jefferson was experiencing. The Philadelphia medical community would turn its greatest scandal into an opportunity to get what eluded them in 1867: a law that applied to the entire state, and mandated the distribution of unclaimed bodies to medical schools.

Pancoast saw the wisdom of McKnight's argument and asked the Philadelphia Anatomical Association (the group that attempted to enforce the 1867 law) to draft a new version of the law. Most recognized that bodies were needed for medical education: it wasn't a question of whether schools should be supplied, but how. The Black Philadelphia press, *The Christian Recorder*, which represented the primary victims of this traffic, agreed:

> Our State authorities…should legislate in regard to this common want; defining what bodies the doctors should have the right to receive. We may be told, however, that this is already the case in not a few of the States. This may possibly be true, but where it is legislated upon at all, it is in such a half-hearted way, that the real necessities of the colleges are but poorly met.[50]

In the following months the association met to write and debate the law. According to Forbes's history of the passage of the anatomy act that he wrote years later, he attended one of the meetings and made a motion that the words "shall give permission" should be replaced by "shall deliver," which would make it required, not optional, to transport the unclaimed dead to medical schools, much to the coroner's chagrin. Forbes had accused the coroner of keeping bodies for his own private anatomy school, which he vehemently denied.[51] Forbes claimed he said that if it was not included, the law "would not be worth the paper on which it was printed."[52] The bill was introduced in the legislature by Senator Joseph E. Reyburn. A petition signed by physicians from medical schools throughout Pennsylvania said of the law, "It will increase the necessary facilities for medical education within this State, and will materially aid in preventing desecration of burial-grounds."[53]

Called "The Act For the promotion of medical science by the distribution and use of unclaimed human bodies for scientific purposes through a board created for that purpose and to prevent unauthorized uses and traffic in human bodies," the law's revisions were significant.[54] It extended the law to the entire state of Pennsylvania, made the distribution of unclaimed bodies mandatory, and created the Anatomical Board of the State of Pennsylvania. Unlike the association created after the 1867 law, the board had legal authority to manage the receipt and distribution of unclaimed bodies to medical schools in the state, and individuals responsible for the dead in public institutions notified the board when they had bodies "required to be buried at the public expense." Gone was the provision in the 1867 law that appeared to allow a person to claim themselves; all unclaimed were eligible for dissection.[55]

The 1883 law only mentioned that family could claim the dead: "no such notice need be given [to the Board] nor shall any such body be delivered if any person claiming to be and satisfying the authorities in charge of said body that he or she is of kindred or is related by marriage to the deceased."[56] Not even friends were allowed to claim them. The law also didn't set a number of hours required to wait before a body was claimed, although it did state that the "dead body shall be held subject to their order in the county where the death occurs for a period not less than twenty-four hours."[57] The effect of the revised provisions was to enforce and expand what the 1867 law sanctioned: the wholesale appropriation of individuals who died in public institutions, primarily the almshouse, the poor and the marginalized.

The debate in the Pennsylvania legislature was similar to those of 1863 and 1867. McKnight pushed for the law in the Senate, where he responded to critics that the law targeted the poor:

> I repeat, Mr. President, this measure is in the interest of the laboring man; it is in the interest of the mechanic; it is in the interest of science; it is in the interest of the poor the world over; it is in the interest of the man who gets torn and lacerated in our mines and workshops, and who is too poor to travel to Philadelphia for his surgical aid. Enact this law, and the young man can go from Allegheny, from Jefferson, and from Armstrong Counties to Philadelphia, and he can legally take the human body, which is the A B C of all medical knowledge, and he can dissect it there, and learn by that means just where each artery is, and where each vein is, and where the different muscles lie and the different relations they sustain to one another, and then he is qualified to return to Allegheny or Jefferson County, locate at the crossroads or in the village, and perform the operations that are so much needed there for the relief of suffering humanity and the suffering poor.[58]

The law was passed after Forbes's trial, which resumed in March, three months after the scandal broke, which allowed tempers to cool from a fever pitch in the aftermath of the crime.[59] The headline in *The Press*'s coverage of the trial was "The Sacredness of Sepulture vs. Anatomical Science."[60] A trial of such a high-profile anatomist was a rare occurrence, but Forbes's predicament in supplying bodies without a sufficient legal source was not. He was in a position that all demonstrators feared, and argued was a legal failure, despite the fact that physicians facilitated and sometimes directly participated in body snatching. This view was expressed in *The Times*:

> It was the narrowness of the Pennsylvania statutes and not any criminal design nor even any carelessness of the right of sepulture that had brought about this scandal; It is all nonsense to profess horror at the discovery that the Jefferson school obtained subjects from graveyards. The Jefferson people were unfortunate in having their source of supply exposed in a rather startling way, but what they have been doing is simply what was necessarily done, a few years ago, before the passage of the anatomy act, and it is easy to understand why the method was revived.[61]

It was an argument that didn't resonate widely with the public. In the wake of the body-snatching scandal of John Scott Harrison, when the Ohio Medical College denied any knowledge of the affair, a newspaper asked, "Is the school any less a party to the felony because it does not know the name of the felon with whom it cooperates?"[62] Few in the Philadelphia medical community believed Forbes had actually committed a crime, and thought that the only reason he was indicted in the first place was that newspapers had whipped up public furor against him.

Forbes was charged with violation of sepulchre and of conspiring with McNamee to plunder Lebanon Cemetery's graves. He pled not guilty to all charges. The jury's job was laid out by the district attorney:

> If that evidence showed that Dr. Forbes had been guilty of opening the graves, or had knowledge of the purpose to violate sepulture, he was as much guilty as any of the four already convicted of that offense. If, however, the bodies were taken to Dr. Forbes, he absolutely ignorant of the source whence they were obtained, but only as provider of material for scientific purposes, exercising due care to that end, then he was entitled to be found not guilty...But if he had

> guilty knowledge, then he was as much an offender against the statute as though he himself had wielded the spade and mattock which violated the tomb.[63]

In other words, Forbes's guilt hinged on what he knew: if he conspired with McNamee, he was guilty, and if he was unaware of where the bodies came from, he was not guilty. But the evidence the jury had to make their decision was primarily the conflicting testimony of Forbes and McNamee: all Forbes had to do was deny the testimony of a convict. Forbes's defense set about destroying McNamee's already thin credibility: "When it comes to a question of oath against oath, which will you believe—the man who has violated law repeatedly, has been a convict, has convicted himself, or the man who has lived uprightly amongst you?"[64] Of course, they also set about reinforcing Forbes's credibility: "It is not likely that Dr. Forbes, the scholar and the gentleman, conspired with a miserable thief like McNamee…to despoil graves of their occupants."[65] In reality, this was a fairly common practice among anatomists.

McNamee testified that he had an arrangement directly with Forbes to supply bodies from Lebanon Cemetery, that he was well aware where the bodies came from. McNamee's wife also testified that she saw Forbes at her husband's business, and when she asked Forbes to bail out McNamee after his arrest, he replied that it was not a good time because of the public clamor over the affair.[66] In his testimony Forbes denied McNamee's claim, and placed the blame on him. Physicians hired middlemen like McNamee so that if something went wrong, they would have plausible deniability, and their supplier could take the blame.

Some of Forbes's explanations were plausible. Forbes said McNamee had the keys because he delivered bodies from legitimate sources, and bodies were brought in at night not because they were illegitimate and transported in secret, but to avoid offending the sensibilities of everyday Philadelphians, although it was a convenient excuse if illegally transporting bodies. Forbes claimed he didn't even see the bodies until they were first embalmed by his assistant and placed in the dissecting room, that he didn't receive them, and that McNamee was paid only for hauling the bodies, which depended on the distance he hauled them from.

But Forbes claimed he never inquired as to the source of the bodies McNamee or anyone else delivered. The defense held that McNamee's testimony could not be trusted, yet the defense's central claim was that Forbes trusted McNamee when he said he hauled the bodies from the prison. This strained credulity. For someone who was so well aware of the challenges facing demonstrators in supplying bodies, and the problems with the 1867 anatomy law he wrote, Forbes's supposed policy of not asking questions was a plea of ignorance, a legal shield. If he didn't ask questions, how would he know if the bodies came from a legitimate source? Forbes was also a member of the association of anatomists set up after the 1867 law and was responsible for the distribution of unclaimed bodies when they could get them, and appointing who would haul them, primarily from the almshouse.[67]

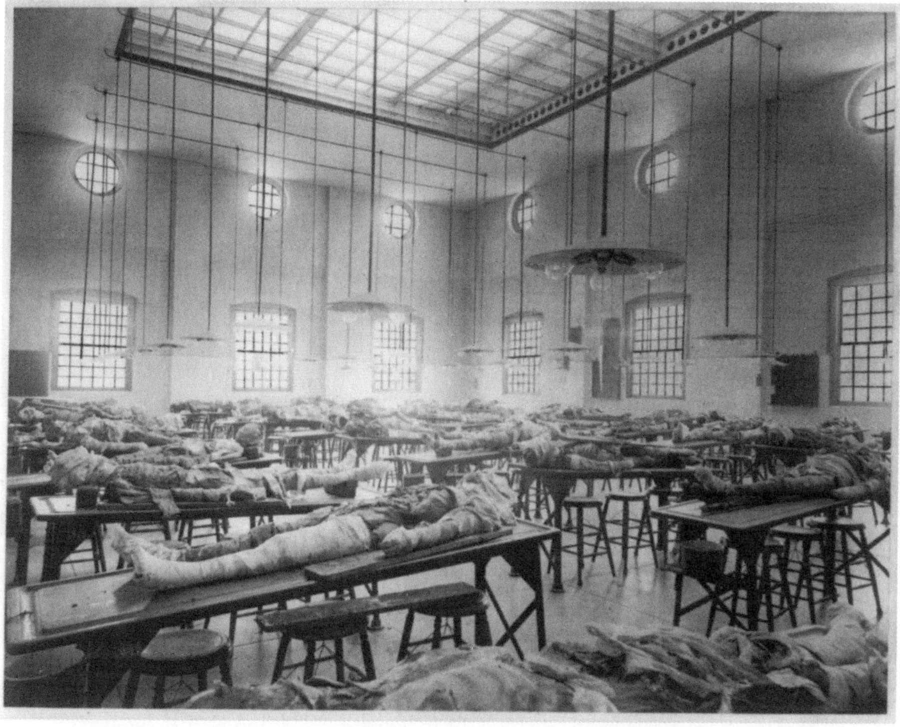

Dissecting room, Jefferson Medical College, 1902. (Library of Congress)

Forbes had to have known how unlikely it was for six people to die at the prison around the same time.

But demonstrators like Forbes had more at stake in securing bodies than just research, instruction, and medical progress: their professional reputation and a source of income. Without bodies Forbes couldn't teach, and without students he wouldn't be paid. Students first paid Forbes 10 dollars to attend his lectures, then paid him a dollar for each of the five "parts" of a body. They were divided into "The head...arms and thorax... and the legs and lower part of the trunk," for a total of five dollars.[68] Forbes paid for the hauling of bodies, but the rest was profit for him to keep. While few likely knew it at the time, at least one of the physician-witnesses called to speak to Forbes's character, David Hayes Agnew, had previously engaged in body snatching himself.[69]

Unlike their speedy verdict for the body snatchers, the jury deliberated for hours before rendering its judgment on Forbes, but when it came he was acquitted. The jury was asked to determine what Forbes knew, but by denying McNamee's testimony and claiming that he never asked about the source of the bodies, the jury let him free either because they believed he told the truth, or that he wasn't required to ask.

The four body snatchers were sentenced soon after, McNamee for eight months, Pillet four months, Levi Chew 18, and Robert Chew two years. As with many cases of body snatching, the perpetrators got off fairly easy, despite the fact that many viewed the crime as an unforgivable violation. Robert's sentence was longer due to the fact that he betrayed the trust he was given to manage the cemetery; he was quickly fired after it was discovered what he did. *The Press*, which first exposed the story, responded to the verdict with silence, despite their frequent coverage before. The work of *The Press*, whose reporting catalyzed these events, unquestionably had value, and exposed crimes against Black Philadelphians, but its sensationalistic coverage that gripped the city soon faded from memory, while the far-reaching legal changes it helped catalyze long outlived it. There were no reported indignation meetings in response to the verdict, but a Black newspaper did respond to the verdict:

> Dr. Forbes, the dealer in cadavers from Lebanon Cemetery, has been tried, and I am sorry to add, has been acquitted. This result was not unexpected when the

> apathy of the trustees is taken in consideration. They made no effort to assist the commonwealth in procuring evidence to convict. Thus far our indignation meetings result only in talk and bluster.[70]

The scandal soon faded from memory, although Forbes also faced civil suits, such as one from the wife of a man buried in Lebanon Cemetery, who sought 20,000 dollars' worth of damages.[71] The result is unknown, but was likely unsuccessful.

In June the governor signed the revised anatomy act. The almshouse reported, "Since the passage of the bill the Almshouse authorities have not buried any of the paupers who have died."[72] Anatomists argued that mandating the distribution of bodies of the poor to medical schools would end body snatching. In actuality, the law achieved the same outcome through legal means. Disinterment was replaced by the legal distribution of bodies of the poor. The point of the law wasn't to punish the poor; they were simply the most vulnerable population to be used for dissection. It was the same logic behind why body snatchers primarily targeted potter's fields and Black cemeteries: they were easier targets.

But body snatching didn't end overnight. In 1884, "A colored man in Camden, New Jersey, has recently been frightening colored people in that city with the idea that he was supplying both living and dead subjects for dissecting rooms. He stated that for living subjects furnished to the Jefferson Medical College he received from twenty-five to thirty dollars, according to their age."[73]

There were false alarms. In 1884 the body of John May, a father who killed his daughter and took his own life in Conshohocken, Pennsylvania, was stolen from his grave in a potter's field in Norristown. What was unusual was the fact that the body was mutilated, and parts that were not wanted—the bowels, liver, lungs, and heart—were placed back in the coffin, and a shovel and a trail of blood were left behind.[74] The body was found in a trunk in the Schuylkill River, weighted with stones inside to hold it down. But it turned out that it was not a case of body snatching at all. Henry A. Fredericks, a railroad employee, and J. B. Weida, a physician who studied medicine in the University of Pennsylvania, had desecrated his grave, to "cut up the body to get the skeleton and a little notoriety also."[75] They turned themselves in, but it appeared doubtful that the two would face harsh punishment.

As the 20th century dawned, and other states passed anatomy acts modeled on Pennsylvania's, body snatching as it was practiced in America before it was even a country gradually ceased.[76] But the law, which appropriated the poor, didn't stop being controversial overnight either. In 1905 an attempt was made to revoke the Pennsylvania act by Henry C. Troxall of the state legislature, to make it so that "by a petition of any 10 taxpayers of the poor district in which the poor person deceased had residence the dead body shall not be given to the Anatomic Board of Pennsylvania."[77] But such attempts failed, and the law survived its challenges.

Lebanon Cemetery was condemned in 1899 and closed in 1903 to make way for the expansion of roads; bodies were reinterred in Eden Cemetery, which still exists today, the oldest Black-owned cemetery in the country.[78] What was the center of Lebanon Cemetery is now a bus stop.[79] In 1903 Frank McNamee met a grim end to his life: he was murdered. He was found "unconscious at Fifth and Walnut streets with his head fractured" and died soon after.[80] It was believed that he was killed by someone upset over the Lebanon Cemetery robbery. Megargee would later be known as the man who "ran down a band of grave robbers."[81] He died in 1905. In 2018 a historical marker for McKnight, who played a crucial role in the passage of the 1883 law, was erected and reads, "A physician turned senator, he coauthored an act in 1883 that established a board to oversee the distribution of unclaimed bodies to medical schools for anatomical study. In effect, it made grave robbery illegal and promoted the advancement of medical science."[82] Forbes was embraced and honored by the medical community after his trial; some even sent money to cover his legal expenses.[83] He became known as the "Father of the Anatomical Act." In 1886 Forbes was promoted, and became Jefferson's professor of anatomy. Upon his death in 1905, Forbes chose to be cremated, a rarity at the time. The keys found on McNamee are in Jefferson's archives today.

In 1903 while digging the foundations for a new addition to Jefferson Hospital, now Jefferson's main building, construction workers discovered two vaults in the ground:

One was 15 feet wide by 20 feet long and 25 feet in height. The only opening was a trap door in the ceiling which communicated with the old dissecting room on the fourth floor by a staircase ladder in the well. It is said to have been built in 1820. The second vault was circular, about 20 feet in diameter and of unknown depth...It is said that these vaults were used formerly to hide the bodies required for dissection, the majority of them having been stolen from graveyards, it being at the time difficult to obtain subjects for that purpose by more legitimate means. In the larger vault several bones were found. The "snatching" of the body of a negro from the old Lebanon Cemetery, at Nineteenth street and Passyunk avenue, in 1880 [1882], led to an investigation and exposure, which resulted in the establishment by the Legislature of the State Anatomical Board, which did away forever with the practice of body snatching.[84]

Afterword

The Legacy of Body Snatching

Show me your cemeteries and I will tell you what kind of people you have.
—BENJAMIN FRANKLIN

Walking through Philadelphia, a city full of life, it's easy to forget that it was built atop the dead. Like other old cities, with land that's been used and reused for hundreds of years, beneath its surface Philadelphia is filled with graves. Some are well remembered. Christ Church Burial Ground in Old City contains the remains of history's most iconic Philadelphian (who was born in Boston): Benjamin Franklin. Visitors and passersby throw pennies on his grave for good luck (Franklin once wrote, "A penny saved is two pence clear," although many mistakenly believe he said, "A penny saved is a penny earned"), which amounts to thousands of dollars that the cemetery collects every year, but not enough to repair the damage the coins contributed to: a crack in Franklin's marble ledger tablet.[1] A successful fundraising campaign in 2016 helped raise enough money for repairs (donations came from the public, the Philadelphia Eagles, and even Bon Jovi).

Other burial places have been long forgotten. In 2013 archeologists confirmed that underneath Weccacoe Playground in South Philadelphia lie the remains of thousands buried in one of the city's first independent cemeteries for free African Americans, the Bethel Burying Ground, of the Mother Bethel African Methodist Episcopal (AME) Church, which dates to the 19th century. A memorial is planned for the site. In 2016 construction workers building a residential complex on Arch Street in Old City unearthed human remains from the First Baptist Church of

Philadelphia burial ground, established in 1707. Archeologists eventually excavated nearly 500 burials, which will be reinterred in Mount Moriah Cemetery; many were destroyed from the construction activity.[2] The bodies were supposed to have been relocated to Mount Moriah Cemetery in 1860, but such relocations were not always fully completed.[3] In 2018 construction workers converting a University of Pennsylvania parking lot into an apartment complex in West Philadelphia discovered that part of the African Friends to Harmony Cemetery, the oldest African American burial ground in that part of the city used in the 19th century, was located on the property.

These discoveries, many of them cemeteries for African Americans, unearthed not just the dead, but the largely forgotten history of their plunder by body snatchers that fueled the rise of medicine and medical education in the city of brotherly love. Even during the peak of body snatching, many believed the practice was a thing of the past: "In the present day, a man may have reasonable hope that his body will be allowed to rest quietly in its appointed grave. But it was not so formerly," according to an 1866 newspaper article.[4] William Shippen Jr., professor of anatomy of the first medical school in the colonies, which would become the University of Pennsylvania, established not just anatomical education in Philadelphia, and America, but how the bodies would be supplied: from the city's marginalized groups. But Black Philadelphians, through force and democratic processes, defended the integrity of their dead, through graveyard patrols, shootouts, and petitions. Anatomy riots broke out, when the public violently expressed their displeasure with the disinterment of the dead by medical men. Secret agreements facilitated the appropriation of the dead from public graveyards, and when they didn't, "professional" body snatchers were hired by doctors to raid them. Cemetery superintendents instituted graveyard defenses, some lethal, to protect the bodies in their care.

The law did little to punish resurrectionists or the doctors who paid for their services, but in 1867 Pennsylvania's first anatomy act legalized a longstanding practice: the appropriation of Philadelphia's poor, primarily from the almshouse. But the law would not reach its full force until 1882, when the theft of bodies from Lebanon Cemetery to Jefferson Medical

College and the scandal that erupted spurred revisions to the law. The 1883 Pennsylvania anatomy act effectively ended body snatching in Pennsylvania by ensuring, with the force of law, that the "unclaimed" would be distributed to medical schools. The cultural meaning of dissection hadn't changed. The dead body has always been infused with meaning, its care or lack of care representing, on one extreme, honor, and on the other, punishment. Dissection was still viewed as a form of punishment, once reserved only for the most reviled in society, but now was reserved only for those who died in public institutions.

Much has changed since the passage of the 1883 anatomy law. The exclusive use of unclaimed bodies in medical schools started to change in the 1950s with the rise of body donation. Once illegal, by then attitudes toward dissection had shifted, from a feared punishment to a viable option for people who wished to have their bodies serve a noble cause, and to reduce their burial costs. In 1968 the Uniform Anatomical Gift Act standardized state-by-state laws on body donation and organ donation. While some question the need for medical students to dissect cadavers given the rise of new technologies, such as interactive software, virtual reality, and 3D models, there's something about the experience of dissecting the body of a real human being, a medical student's "first patient," that can't be replicated any other way, and remains an invaluable rite of passage. However, the availability of alternative ways to learn anatomy means that it's unlikely doctors or medical students will feel the need to return to their past body-snatching ways.

Medicine of course has also changed, not just in terms of treatments, but culture. Medical paternalism—that the doctor knows best and decides what's in the patient's best interest—has given way to informed consent—that patients make decisions about their health with the information provided to them by their doctor. Instead of seeing bodies for dissection as purely objects to be studied, they're more likely to be seen as human beings who selflessly gave their bodies to science; instead of clinical detachment, clinical empathy is taught in medical schools, which offers a more nuanced, humane approach to interacting with patients. The profession is now reckoning with its dark past more than it ever has before, which body snatching was a part of.

Much has changed, but one thing has stayed the same: Pennsylvania's 1883 anatomy act. The law has been amended since, but it's still in effect today. What was once called the Anatomical Board of the State of Pennsylvania has been renamed the Humanity Gifts Registry (HGR), a non-profit agency that distributes donated bodies to Pennsylvania medical schools, such as the University of Pennsylvania and Jefferson, as well as dental schools. All body donations in the state go through the HGR, which distributes them, just as it did in the 19th century. Every year a "Celebration of Remembrance" is held where students and families and friends of donors are honored for their contribution to science, now a common practice in medical schools across the country. Bodies are cremated after study and buried or returned to the families of the deceased. A form is available on their website to become a donor, which requires two witnesses.

Around 20,000 Americans donate their bodies to science annually. Most donors are also white, likely because of lower levels of trust among minority groups given the medical community's long history of exploitation. While the majority of bodies dissected in medical schools are donated, and the involuntary dissection of marginalized groups has mostly given way to voluntary dissection of donors, the unclaimed—without consent—are still dissected today, although it varies from state to state and even school to school.

As per Pennsylvania's 1883 anatomy law, a body is considered unclaimed after 36 hours, after which it is kept in storage for three months, cremated, and stored for 10 years; families can claim the cremains for free.[5] Most bodies are unclaimed for the same reason they were unclaimed in the 19th century: the families of the deceased couldn't afford to claim them.[6] In 1994 the Philadelphia Medical Examiner's Office transported 36 unclaimed bodies to a school without the consent of families.[7] In 2016 New York banned the dissection of unclaimed bodies without consent of the deceased's family. The use of unclaimed bodies is legal in most states, but there is little data about the practice. In 2024 it was discovered that a Texas medical school received unclaimed bodies for years, without notifying families, and leased the bodies out for medical research.

Like body donation, organ donation is also regulated by the Uniform Anatomical Gift Act. But surprisingly, buying and selling human remains is legal in most states, including Pennsylvania. Non-transplant tissue banks, referred to by critics as "body brokers," accept donations of bodies with the consent of the deceased or their family. The companies pay for the body's cremation, but profit from selling body parts for research and instruction with little federal oversight. Federal legislation has been proposed to regulate this trade, but it has not been passed. This legal gray area also facilitates the "oddities" trade.

In 2023 the U.S. Attorney's Office for the Middle District of Pennsylvania indicted Harvard Medical School's morgue manager for selling human remains stolen from Harvard donors across the country, and others, including two Pennsylvanians, for buying and reselling them. While a state agency handles body donations in Pennsylvania, medical schools in other states can directly receive donations. Before cremating the bodies after students were done dissecting them, for years the morgue manager used his position to steal parts from bodies to sell online, which he shipped through USPS to states like Pennsylvania; some of his buyers visited the morgue to pick the parts they wanted.

In one PayPal transaction, one of the people charged from West Lawn, Pennsylvania, sent 200 dollars to the morgue manager's wife, who participated in the scheme, with the following message: "braiiiiiins."[8] Another person indicted from Salem, Massachusetts, shipped human skin to a Pennsylvanian from Bloomsburg, for him to tan and make into leather, who accepted more skin as payment. With no laws against buying and selling human remains, they were charged with conspiring to transport stolen goods across state lines, just as body snatchers of the past were charged with other crimes when no statutes banned the practice.[9] One of the Pennsylvanians was sentenced to two years on probation, and others are still awaiting trial. Instead of buying and selling whole bodies for medical education, body parts are bought and sold in the "oddities" trade for macabre personal collections. Much of this trade is openly conducted online, in conventions and shops, which is legal in most states, as long as the remains aren't stolen. But where the specimens bought and sold are sourced from is an open question, and how one can verify they aren't stolen, is an open question. The vast majority of people, both past and present, would probably have a problem with their skull being displayed on someone's mantel as a macabre decoration.

Museums and universities store and display collections of human remains, some of which were obtained through body snatching at a time when informed consent wasn't practiced. In 2024 the University of Pennsylvania's Penn Museum interred the skulls of 19 Black Philadelphians from its Morton Cranial Collection in Eden Cemetery, a historic Black cemetery in Pennsylvania. Some of the bones were taken by Samuel George Morton, a Philadelphia doctor, from the city's Blockley Almshouse—some of whom were formerly enslaved—and used to support scientific racism, the pseudoscientific belief that there is a hierarchy of human races, with white people on top.[10] The bottom of a memorial stone placed in the cemetery for the skulls reads: "May they finally have peace." The bones were previously displayed in a classroom in the museum until protests by students in 2020. The Penn Museum no longer exhibits "exposed" human remains, in which parts of the body are visible (it still displays mummies and other enclosed bodies).[11]

The Mütter Museum, a Philadelphia medical history museum, has come under intense scrutiny from people who believe the remains it displays without consent, some of which were obtained through body snatching, should not be displayed, and others who believe that not doing so would be a disservice, that the collection should remain available for the public and researchers to understand the painful past of medical exploitation (a small percentage of the museum's collection was obtained with the consent of donors).[12] There is a worldwide debate surrounding the display and treatment of human remains. Is it ethical to display remains obtained without the permission of the deceased? Can such human remains be respectfully displayed? What would that look like? Does the display of such remains repeat past abuses, or does their educational and research value outweigh other considerations? Who should decide?

Institutions like the Penn Museum have sought the input of ancestral communities in deciding how to handle its Morton Cranial Collection. The Mütter Museum is conducting a review of its collection and gathering feedback to shape the museum's future. In a shifting ethical landscape, institutions are attempting to seek input to decide how to move forward, with varying levels of success. There are no easy answers, only hard questions that will continue to be fiercely debated.

Philadelphia's dominance in medicine and medical education has faded since its peak in the 19th century, but today one in six of the nation's doctors are educated in the city, and its hospitals and medical schools are world renowned. We can only speculate what the world would be like today if body snatching had never been practiced, but regardless, we are living with the consequences, for better and worse.

The medical community's exploitation of minority groups, including body snatching, the distrust it engendered, and the racism and bias that pervaded medical practice still impacts health outcomes today. Many if not most anatomy acts passed in the 19th or early 20th centuries are still in force today, some of which still appropriate the unclaimed for dissection. The International Federation of Associations of Anatomists, the American Association for Anatomy, and the American Medical Association recommend exclusively using donated bodies for dissection. The number of unclaimed bodies used to learn anatomy has even been increasing in some areas, such as Texas. Body parts are legally bought and sold in a largely unregulated market, for personal collections or research and instruction. While legal, it's a system ripe for abuse that demands greater oversight. Collections obtained through body snatching are still stored or displayed in museums and universities today, and spark debates surrounding the ethical treatment of human remains. The history of body snatching is still being unearthed, from archives, newspapers, medical journals, and other sources. Every American city with medical schools has a story to tell about the grave dealings of the body snatchers, none more so than Philadelphia, and the legacy of this strange time when crime and medicine collided in America's first capital city lives on.

Appendix

While Pennsylvania's anatomy law was passed in 1883 and has been amended since, the law is still in effect today. It is the only entity in the state that has the power to receive and distribute the dead to medical schools. Unlike when the law was passed, the majority of bodies distributed in the state in the present day are voluntarily donated, not unclaimed.

Pennsylvania's 1883 anatomy law reads:

> AN ACT
> For the promotion of medical science by the distribution and use of unclaimed human bodies for scientific purposes through a board created for that purpose and to prevent unauthorized uses and traffic in human bodies.
>
> SECTION 1. *Be it enacted, etc.*, That the professors of anatomy, the professors of surgery, the demonstrators of anatomy and the demonstrators of surgery of the medical and dental schools and colleges of this Commonwealth, which are now or may hereafter become incorporated, together with one representative from each of the unincorporated schools of anatomy or practical surgery, within this Commonwealth, in which there are from time to time, at the time of the appointment of such representatives, shall be not less than five scholars, shall be and hereby are constituted a board for the distribution and delivery of dead human bodies, hereinafter described, to and among such persons as, under the provisions of this act, are entitled thereto. The professor of anatomy in the University of Pennsylvania, at Philadelphia, shall call a meeting of said board for organization at a time and place to be fixed by him within thirty days after the passage of this act. The said board shall have full power to establish rules and regulations for its government, and to appoint and remove proper officers, and shall keep full and complete minutes of its transactions; and records shall also be kept under its direction of all bodies received and distributed by said board, and of the persons to whom the same may be distributed, which minutes and records shall be open

at all times to the inspection of each member of said board, and of any district attorney of any county within this Commonwealth.

SECTION 2. All public officers, agents and servants, and all officers, agents and servants of any and every county, city, township, borough, district and other municipality, and of any and every alms-house, prison, morgue, hospital, or other public institution having charge or control over dead human bodies, required to be buried at the public expense, are hereby required to notify the said board of distribution or [*sic*] such person or persons as may, from time to time, be designated by said board or its duly authorized officer or agent, whenever any such body or bodies come to his or their possession, charge or control, and shall, without fee or reward, deliver such body or bodies, and permit and suffer the said board and its agents, and the physicians and surgeons from time to time designated by them, who may comply with the provisions of this act, to take and remove all such bodies to be used within this State for the advancement of medical science, but no such notice need be given nor shall any such body be delivered if any person claiming to be and satisfying the authorities in charge of said body that he or she is of kindred or is related by marriage to the deceased, shall claim the said body for burial, but it shall be surrendered for interment, nor shall the notice be given or body delivered if such deceased person was a traveler who died suddenly, in which case the said body shall be buried.

SECTION 3. The said board or their duly authorized agent may take and receive such bodies so delivered as aforesaid, and shall, upon receiving them, distribute and deliver them to and among the schools, colleges, physicians and surgeons aforesaid, in manner following: Those bodies needed for lectures and demonstrations by the said schools and colleges incorporated and unincorporated shall first be supplied, the remaining bodies shall then be distributed proportionately and equitably, preference being given to said schools and colleges, the number assigned to each to be based upon the number of students in each dissecting or operative surgery class which number shall be reported to the board at such time as it may direct. Instead of receiving and delivering said bodies themselves, or through their agents or servants, the board of distribution may, from time to time, either directly or by their authorized officer or agent, designate physicians and surgeons who shall receive them, and the number which each shall receive: *Provided always however*, That schools and colleges incorporated and unincorporated, and physicians or surgeons of the county where the death of the person or such person described takes place, shall be preferred to all others: *And provided also*, That for this purpose such dead body shall be held subject to their order in the county where the death occurs for a period not less than twenty-four hours.

SECTION 4. The said board may employ a carrier or carriers for the conveyance of said bodies, which shall be well enclosed within a suitable encasement, and carefully deposited free from public observation. Said carrier shall obtain receipts by name, or if the person be unknown by a description of each body delivered by him, and shall deposit said receipt with the secretary of the said board.

SECTION 5. No school, college, physician or surgeon shall be allowed or permitted to receive any such body or bodies until a bond shall have been given to the Commonwealth by such physician or surgeon, or by or in [*sic*] behalf of such school or college, to be approved by the prothonotary of the court of common pleas in and for the county in which such physician or surgeon shall reside, or in which such school or college may be situate [*sic*], and to be filed in the office of said prothonotary, which bond shall be in the penal sum of one thousand dollars, conditioned that all such bodies which the said physician or surgeon, or the said school or college shall receive thereafter shall be used only for the promotion of medical science within this State, and whosoever shall sell or buy such body or bodies, or in any way traffic in the same, or shall transmit or convey or cause to procure to be transmitted or conveyed said body or bodies, to any place outside of this State, shall be deemed guilty of a misdemeanor, and shall on conviction, be liable to a fine not exceeding two hundred dollars, or be imprisoned for a term not exceeding one year.

SECTION 6. Neither the Commonwealth nor any county or municipality, nor any officer, agent or servant thereof, shall be at any expense by reason of the delivery or distribution of any such body, but all the expenses thereof and of said board of distribution shall be paid by those receiving the bodies, in such manner as may be specified by said board of distribution, or otherwise agreed upon.

SECTION 7. That any person having duties enjoined upon him by the provisions of this act who shall neglect, refuse or omit to perform the same as hereby required, shall on conviction thereof, be liable to a fine of not less than one hundred nor more than five hundred dollars for each offense.

SECTION 8. That all acts or parts of acts inconsistent with this act be and the same are hereby repealed.

APPROVED—The 13th day of June, A. D. 1883. ROBT. E. PATTISON, *Governor.*[1]

Endnotes

Note: all hyperlinks referenced in the endnotes were accessed between October 2022 and January 2025.

Introduction: Death, Disinterment, and Dissection in Philadelphia

1 Arthur Wentworth Eaton, *Funny Epitaphs* (Boston: The Mutual Book Company, 1902), 28, Project Gutenberg.

2 This case of body snatching, the most infamous in Philadelphia history, is the subject of chapter seven.

3 William Hunter, *Two Introductory Lectures, Delivered by Dr. William Hunter* (London: Printed by Order of the Trustees, for J. Johnson, No. 72, St. Paul's Church-Yard, 1784), 67, Wellcome Collection.

4 Ruth Richardson, "A Necessary Inhumanity?" *Journal of Medical Ethics* 26, no. 6 (December 2000): 104–6, Gale.

5 Lindsey Fitzharris, *The Butchering Art* (New York: Scientific American/Farrar, Straus and Giroux, 2017), 10.

6 "Chapter 7: Eminent Jefferson Professors," 231–386, in *Legend and Lore: Jefferson Medical College. Paper 8* (2009), 259, http://jdc.jefferson.edu/savacool/8.

7 "The Secret Lives of Cadavers: How Lifeless Bodies Become Life-Saving Tools," *National Geographic*, last modified July 29, 2016, https://www.nationalgeographic.com/science/article/body-donation-cadavers-anatomy-medical-education?loggedin=true&rnd=1705108502113.

8 *Daily Patriot and Union* (Harrisburg, PA), March 30, 1861, Pennsylvania Newspaper Archive, quoted in Steven Robert Wilf, "Anatomy and Punishment in Late Eighteenth-Century New York," *Journal of Social History* 22, no. 3 (Spring 1989): 509, JSTOR.

9 Edward H. Dixon, "Scenes in a Medical Student's Life—Resurrectionizing," *Scalpel: An Entirely Original Quarterly Expositor of the Laws of Health, and Abuses of Medicine and Domestic Life* 7 (1855): 94, Gale.

10 "Black Philadelphians in the Samuel George Morton Cranial Collection," Penn Program on Race, Science & Society, last modified February 15, 2021, https://prss.sas.upenn.edu/projects/penn-medicines-role/black-philadelphians-samuel-george-morton-cranial-collection.
11 James O. Breeden, "Body Snatchers and Anatomy Professors: Medical Education in Nineteenth-Century Virginia," *The Virginia Magazine of History and Biography* 83, no. 3 (July 1975): 321, JSTOR.
12 Dr. Frederick C. Waite, "Grave Robbing in New England," *Bulletin of the Medical Library Association* 33, no. 3 (July 1945): 272–73.
13 "Holy Experiment," The Encyclopedia of Greater Philadelphia, accessed September 1, 2024, https://philadelphiaencyclopedia.org/themes/holy-experiment-2/.
14 Stephen Nepa, "Cemeteries," The Encyclopedia of Greater Philadelphia, accessed September 1, 2024, https://philadelphiaencyclopedia.org/essays/cemeteries/.
15 Thomas W. Laqueur, *The Work of the Dead: A Cultural History of Mortal Remains* (Princeton and Oxford: Princeton University Press, 2015), 10.
16 Robert Halliday, "The Roadside Burial of Suicides: An East Anglian Study," *Folklore* 121, no. 1 (April 2010): 81–93, JSTOR.
17 Venetia M. Guerrasio, "Dissecting the Pennsylvania Anatomy Act: Laws, Bodies, and Science, 1880–1960," (PhD diss., University of New Hampshire, Durham, 2007), 4, University of New Hampshire Scholars Repository (376).

Chapter 1: "Now and Then One From the Potter's Field": Washington Square and America's First Medical School

1 T. S. Sozinsky, "Grave-Robbing and Dissection," *The Penn Monthly* 10 (January–December 1879): 217, HathiTrust.
2 Nicholas A. Basbanes, *A Gentle Madness: Bibliophiles, Bibliomanes, and the Eternal Passion for Books* (New York: Henry Holt and Company, 1995), 130.
3 George W. Norris, *The Early History of Medicine in Philadelphia* (Philadelphia: Collins Printing House, 1886), 99, Internet Archive.
4 Francis R. Packard, "Early Methods of Medical Education in North America," *The Journal of the American Medical Association* XXXII, no. 12 (March 1899): 636, Internet Archive.
5 Packard, "Early Methods of Medical Education in North America," 636.
6 Basbanes, *A Gentle Madness*, 130.
7 James Thacher, *American Medical Biography: Or Memoirs of Eminent Physicians Who Have Flourished in America*, Vol. I (Boston: Richardson & Lord and Cottons & Barnard, 1828), 52, Internet Archive.
8 "Forbes Expedition," George Washington's Mount Vernon, accessed September 6, 2024, https://www.mountvernon.org/library/digitalhistory/digital-encyclopedia/article/forbes-expedition/.

9 Howard A. Kelly and Walter L. Burrage, *American Medical Biographies* (Baltimore: The Norman, Remington Company, 1920), 1045–46, Internet Archive.
10 Ibid., 1045.
11 John Fanning Watson, *Annals of Philadelphia and Pennsylvania, In the Olden Time*, Vol. II (self-pub., 1850), 378, Internet Archive.
12 Betsy Copping Corner, *William Shippen, Jr., Pioneer in American Medical Education* (Philadelphia: American Philosophical Society, 1951), 8, HathiTrust.
13 "Galen," Britannica, last modified August 21, 2024, https://www.britannica.com/biography/Galen.
14 Charles McRae, *Fathers of Biology* (London: Percival & Co, 1890), 68, Project Gutenberg.
15 Don K. Nakayama, "Guild Rivalries Between Barbers and Surgeons in Medieval London and England," *The American Surgeon* 89, no. 12 (December 2023): 1, Sage Journals.
16 Roderick E. McGrew, *Encyclopedia of Medical History* (New York: McGraw-Hill Book Company, 1985), 30, Internet Archive.
17 Ibid., 30–31.
18 Wendy Moore, *The Knife Man: Blood, Body Snatching, and the Birth of Modern Surgery* (New York: Broadway Books, 2005), 27.
19 Corner, *William Shippen, Jr., Pioneer in American Medical Education*, 8.
20 Ibid., 25.
21 Peter Linebaugh, "The Tyburn Riot Against the Surgeons," in *Albion's Fatal Tree: Crime and Society in Eighteenth-Century England* (London: Verso, 2011), 81.
22 "Murder Act 1751," Wikisource, accessed September 25, 2024, https://en.wikisource.org/wiki/Murder_Act_1751.
23 Michael Sappol, *A Traffic of Dead Bodies: Anatomy and Embodied Social Identity in Nineteenth-Century America* (Princeton: Princeton University Press, 2002), 101.
24 Wilf, "Anatomy and Punishment in Late Eighteenth-Century New York," 510.
25 "Ordinary of Newgate's Account July 1752," Old Bailey Proceedings Online, accessed September 25, 2024, https://www.oldbaileyonline.org/record/OA17520702.
26 Moore, *The Knife Man*, 37.
27 James Blake Bailey, *The Diary of a Resurrectionist 1811–1812* (London: Swan Sonnenschein & Co., Lim, 1896), 150, Project Gutenberg.
28 Hubert Cole, *Things for the Surgeon: A History of the Resurrection Men* (London: Heinemann, 1964), 15, Internet Archive.
29 Julia Bess Frank, "Body Snatching: A Grave Medical Problem," *The Yale Journal of Biology and Medicine* 49 (1976): 402, PubMed.
30 "Resurrecting the Body Snatchers: The Halloween Edition," Dr. Lindsey Fitzharris, accessed September 25, 2024, https://drlindseyfitzharris.com/resurrecting-the-body-snatchers-the-halloween-edition/.
31 "Statement on the Skeleton of Charles Byrne from the Board of Trustees of the Hunterian Collection," Hunterian Museum, last modified January 11, 2023, https://hunterianmuseum.org/news/statement-on-the-skeleton-of-charles-byrne-from-the-board-of-trustees-of-the-hunterian-collection.

32 Moore, *The Knife Man*, 37.
33 Corner, *William Shippen, Jr., Pioneer in American Medical Education*, 67.
34 "From Benjamin Franklin to Jacques Barbeu-Dubourg, 28 July 1768," Founders Online, accessed September 25, 2024, https://founders.archives.gov/documents/Franklin/01-15-02-0098.
35 Betsy Copping Corner, "Day Book of an Education: William Shippen's Student Days in London (1759–1760) and His Subsequent Career," *Proceedings of the American Philosophical Society* 94, no. 2 (April 1950): 132, JSTOR.
36 "Craven Street Bones," Benjamin Franklin House, accessed September 25, 2024, https://benjaminfranklinhouse.org/the-house-benjamin-franklin/craven-street-bones/.
37 "A Brief History of Benjamin Franklin's Residences on Craven Street, London: 1757–1775," Journal of the American Revolution, last modified March 23, 2016, https://allthingsliberty.com/2016/03/a-brief-history-of-benjamin-franklins-residences-on-craven-street-london-1757-1775/.
38 Suzanne M. Shultz, *Body Snatching: The Robbing of Graves for the Education of Physicians in Early Nineteenth Century America* (Jefferson: McFarland & Company, 1992), 27.
39 Corner, *William Shippen, Jr., Pioneer in American Medical Education*, 80.
40 Betsy Copping Corner, "Dr. John Fothergill and the American Colonies," *Quaker History* 52, no. 2 (Autumn 1963): 79, JSTOR.
41 Corner, *William Shippen, Jr., Pioneer in American Medical Education*, 98.
42 *The Pennsylvania Gazette* (Philadelphia, PA), November 11, 1762, History Commons.
43 Sappol, *A Traffic of Dead Bodies*, 70.
44 Whitfield J. Bell, Jr., *The Colonial Physician & Other Essays* (New York: Science History Publications, 1975), 216.
45 Lawrence C. Parish and Thomas N. Haviland, "Surgeons' Hall—The Story of the First Medical-School Building in the United States," *The New England Journal of Medicine* 273, no. 19 (1965): 1021.
46 Stephen Fried, *Rush: Revolution, Madness, and the Visionary Doctor Who Became a Founding Father* (New York: Crown, 2018), 38.
47 George W. Corner, *Two Centuries of Medicine: A History of the School of Medicine, University of Pennsylvania* (Philadelphia: J. B. Lippincott Company, 1965), 12.
48 *The Pennsylvania Gazette* (Philadelphia, PA), November 11, 1762, History Commons.
49 *The Pennsylvania Gazette* (Philadelphia, PA), December 2, 1762, History Commons.
50 Watson, *Annals of Philadelphia and Pennsylvania, In the Olden Time*, Vol. II, 379.
51 Ibid.
52 Ibid.
53 Ibid.
54 "In the Ghostly Old Times," *The Hazleton Sentinel* (Hazleton, Pennsylvania), August 7, 1906, Newspapers.com.
55 Watson, *Annals of Philadelphia and Pennsylvania, In the Olden Time*, Vol. II, 379.
56 Ibid., 379–80.

57 Thomas Hood, "Mary's Ghost. A Pathetic Ballad," Wikisource, accessed December 1, 2024, https://en.wikisource.org/wiki/Mary%27s Ghost. A_Pathetic_Ballad.
58 Edward Mussey Hartwell, "The Hindrances to Anatomical Study in the United States, Including a Special Record of the Struggles of Our Early Anatomical Teachers," in *Annals of Anatomy and Surgery: The Journal of the Anatomical and Surgical Society*, ed. Lewis S. Pilcher and George R. Fowler (Brooklyn: 1881), 216, HathiTrust.
59 Corner, *William Shippen, Jr., Pioneer in American Medical Education*, 98.
60 Corner, *Two Centuries of Medicine*, 22; John Morgan, *A Discourse upon the Institution of Medical Schools in America* (Philadelphia: Printed and sold by William Bradford, 1765), 35, PubMed.
61 Corner, *William Shippen, Jr., Pioneer in American Medical Education*, 110.
62 *The Pennsylvania Gazette* (Philadelphia, PA), September 26, 1765, History Commons.
63 Suzanne M. Shultz, "Colonial Medical Practice: A Case Study of Thomas Cadwalader (1708–1779)," *Journal of Medical Biography* 3 (August 1995): 133, Sage.
64 Whitfield J. Bell Jr., "Medical Practice in Colonial America," *Bulletin of the History of Medicine* 31, no. 5 (September–October 1957): 442.
65 Sappol, *A Traffic of Dead Bodies*, 47–48.
66 *The Pennsylvania Gazette* (Philadelphia, PA), September 26, 1765, History Commons.
67 Timothy J. Hayburn, "Who Should Die?: The Evolution of Capital Punishment in Pennsylvania, 1681–1794," (PhD diss., Lehigh University, 2011), 213, ProQuest.
68 *The Pennsylvania Gazette* (Philadelphia, PA), September 26, 1765, History Commons.
69 "Green Country Town," The Encyclopedia of Greater Philadelphia, accessed September 29, 2024, https://philadelphiaencyclopedia.org/themes/green-country-town/.
70 "Cemeteries," The Encyclopedia of Greater Philadelphia, accessed September 29, 2024, https://philadelphiaencyclopedia.org/essays/cemeteries/.
71 J. Thomas Scharf and Thompson Westcott, *History of Philadelphia. 1609–1884*, Vol. III (Philadelphia: L. H. Everts & Co., 1884), 2355, Internet Archive.
72 John Fanning Watson, *Annals of Philadelphia and Pennsylvania, In the Olden Time*, Vol. I (self-pub., 1884), 406, Internet Archive.
73 "In the Ghostly Old Times," *The Hazleton Sentinel* (Hazleton, Pennsylvania), August 7, 1906, Newspapers.com.
74 Erik R. Seeman, *Death in the New World: Cross-Cultural Encounters, 1492–1800* (Philadelphia: University of Pennsylvania Press, 2010), 43; Aaron Vickers Wunsch, "Parceling the Picturesque: 'Rural' Cemeteries and Urban Context in Nineteenth-Century Philadelphia," (PhD diss., University of California, 2009), 6, eScholarship.
75 Wunsch, "Parceling the Picturesque," 7.
76 Scharf and Westcott, *History of Philadelphia. 1609–1884*, Vol. III, 2356.
77 Gary Laderman, *The Sacred Remains: American Attitudes Toward Death, 1799–1883* (New Haven: Yale University Press, 1996), 27–28.

78 Ibid., 28.
79 Simon P. Newman, *Embodied History: The Lives of the Poor in Early Philadelphia* (Philadelphia: University of Pennsylvania Press, 2003), 61.
80 Wunsch, "Parceling the Picturesque: 'Rural' Cemeteries and Urban Context in Nineteenth-Century Philadelphia," 5.
81 Ruth Richardson, *Death, Dissection and the Destitute* (Chicago: The University of Chicago Press, 2000), 17–18.
82 Seeman, *Death in the New World,* 24–25.
83 "Cemeteries," The Encyclopedia of Greater Philadelphia, accessed September 30, 2024, https://philadelphiaencyclopedia.org/archive/cemeteries/.
84 Seeman, *Death in the New World,* 24.
85 Ibid., 15.
86 Ibid., 12.
87 Hartwell, "The Hindrances to Anatomical Study in the United States," 217.
88 Francis Hopkinson, *An Oration, Which Might Have Been Delivered to the Students in Anatomy, On the Late Rupture Between the Two Schools in this City* (Philadelphia: T. Dobson and T. Lang, 1789), 6, National Library of Medicine.
89 Roger D. Simon, *Philadelphia: A Brief History* (Philadelphia: Temple University Press, 2017), 5; Newman, *Embodied History: The Lives of the Poor in Early Philadelphia,* 105; Jacob Mordecai, "Addenda to Watson's Annals of Philadelphia," *The Pennsylvania Magazine of History and Biography* 98, no. 2 (1974): 141, JSTOR.
90 Erik R. Seeman, *Speaking with the Dead in Early America* (Philadelphia: University of Pennsylvania Press, 2019), 120–21.
91 Ibid., 121.
92 J. T. Headley, *The Great Riots of New York 1712 to 1873: Including a Full and Complete Account of the Four Days' Draft Riot of 1863* (New York: E. B. Treat, 1873), Project Gutenberg.
93 Ibid.
94 Whitfield J. Bell, Jr., "Doctors' Riot, New York, 1788," *Bulletin of the New York Academy of Medicine* 47, no. 12 (December 1971): 1503, PubMed.
95 *The Pennsylvania Gazette* (Philadelphia, PA), January 11, 1770, History Commons.
96 Ibid.
97 Hayburn, "Who Should Die?" 232.
98 *The Pennsylvania Gazette* (Philadelphia, PA), April 26, 1770 and November 8, 1770.
99 "John Adams to Abigail Adams, 13 April 1777," Founders Online, accessed September 30, 2024, https://founders.archives.gov/documents/Adams/04-02-02-0158.
100 "British Occupation of Philadelphia," The Encyclopedia of Greater Philadelphia, accessed September 30, 2024, https://philadelphiaencyclopedia.org/essays/british-occupation-of-philadelphia/.
101 "John Morgan vs. William Shippen: The Battle that Defined the Continental Medical Department," Journal of the American Revolution, accessed October 3,

2024, https://allthingsliberty.com/2020/01/john-morgan-vs-william-shippen-the-battle-that-defined-the-medical-department/.

102 Ibid.

103 Whitfield J. Bell, Jr., "The Court Martial of Dr. William Shippen, Jr., 1780," *Journal of the History of Medicine and Allied Sciences* 19, no. 3 (July 1964): 220, JSTOR.

104 "From George Washington to William Shippen, Jr., 6 February 1777," Founders Online, accessed September 30, 2024, https://founders.archives.gov/documents/Washington/03-08-02-0281.

105 William Shippen Jr. to Thomas Lee Shippen, December 18, 1787, Shippen Family Papers, Library of Congress, Washington, D.C.

106 "In the Ghostly Old Times," *The Hazleton Sentinel* (Hazleton, Pennsylvania), Aug. 7, 1906, Newspapers.com.

107 Francis Hopkinson, *An Oration, Which Might Have Been Delivered to the Students in Anatomy*, 8.

108 William Shippen Jr. to Thomas Lee Shippen, December 18, 1787, Shippen Family Papers, Library of Congress, Washington, D.C.

109 William Shippen Jr. to Thomas Lee Shippen, December 31, 1787, Shippen Family Papers, Library of Congress, Washington, D.C.

110 "Police Department (Philadelphia)," The Encyclopedia of Greater Philadelphia, accessed September 30, 2024, https://philadelphiaencyclopedia.org/essays/police-department-philadelphia/.

111 Gary B. Nash and Jean R. Soderlund, *Freedom By Degrees: Emancipation in Pennsylvania and Its Aftermath* (New York: Oxford University Press, 1991), 111.

112 Ibid., 9; Charles L. Blockson, *African Americans in Pennsylvania: Above Ground and Underground* (Harrisburg: Regent Publishing Services, 2001), 13.

113 Kimberly A. Morrell, "Phase IB Archaeological Investigations of the Mother Bethel Burying Ground, 1810–Circa 1864," accessed September 30, 2024, https://bethelburyinggroundproject.com/wp-content/uploads/2015/01/2.pdf.

114 "Free African Society," The Encyclopedia of Greater Philadelphia, accessed September 30, 2024, https://philadelphiaencyclopedia.org/archive/free-african-society/.

115 Morrell, "Phase IB Archaeological Investigations of the Mother Bethel Burying Ground, 1810–Circa 1864."

116 John Francis Marion, *Philadelphia Medica* (Harrisburg: SmithKline Corporation, 1975), 97.

117 Robert J. Hunter, *The Origin of the Philadelphia General Hospital Blockley Division* (Philadelphia: The Rittenhouse Press, 1955), 35.

118 Hayburn, "Who Should Die?" 233.

119 *The Pennsylvania Mercury, and Universal Advertiser* (Philadelphia, PA), March 8, 1788.

120 Madlen Read, "Perspective: Haunted Philadelphia," *The Daily Pennsylvanian*, October 29, 2002, https://www.thedp.com/article/2002/10/perspective_haunted_philadelphia.

121 Lawrence C. Parish and Thomas N. Haviland, "Surgeons' Hall—The Story of the First Medical-School Building in the United States," 1022.

122 Corner, *Two Centuries of Medicine*, 50.
123 Ibid.
124 "From George Washington to Tobias Lear, 25 September 1793," Founders Online, accessed September 30, 2024, https://founders.archives.gov/documents/Washington/05-14-02-0095.
125 Marion, *Philadelphia Medica*, 23.

Chapter 2: "Board of Buzzards": Dissecting the Destitute at Blockley Almshouse

1 David Hayes Agnew, Alfred Stille, Lewis P. Bush, Charles K. Mills, and Roland G. Curtin, *History and Reminiscences of the Philadelphia Almshouse and Philadelphia Hospital* (Philadelphia: Detre & Blackburn, 1890), 41, HathiTrust.
2 Thomas A. Crist, Douglas B. Mooney, and Kimberly A. Morrell, "'The Mangled Remains of What Had Been Humanity': Evidence of Autopsy and Dissection at Philadelphia's Blockley Almshouse, 1835–1895," in *The Bioarchaeology of Dissection and Autopsy in the United States*, ed. Kenneth C. Nystrom (Switzerland: Springer, 2017), 266–67.
3 Faye Flam, "Anatomy's Graveyard," *Philadelphia Inquirer* (Philadelphia, PA), May 7, 2007, https://www.inquirer.com/philly/health/20070507_Anatomys_graveyard.html.
4 "Almshouses (Poorhouses)," The Encyclopedia of Greater Philadelphia, accessed October 30, 2024, https://philadelphiaencyclopedia.org/essays/almshouses-poorhouses/.
5 *The Pennsylvania Gazette* (Philadelphia, PA), May 29, 1776, History Commons.
6 Leonard Warren, *Joseph Leidy: The Last Man Who Knew Everything* (New Haven: Yale University Press, 1998), 26.
7 Simon Baatz, "'A Very Diffused Disposition': Dissecting Schools in Philadelphia, 1823–1825," *The Pennsylvania Magazine of History and Biography* 108, no. 2 (1984): 206, JSTOR; "City of Medicine," The Encyclopedia of Greater Philadelphia, accessed October 12, 2024, https://philadelphiaencyclopedia.org/themes/city-of-medicine/#:~:text=For%20most%20of%20the%20nineteenth,as%20a%20city%20of%20medicine.
8 "Medical Schools," *Register and Library of Medical and Chirurgical Science* I, no. 3 (October 10, 1833): 25–26, EBSCOhost.
9 Sappol, *A Traffic of Dead Bodies*, 2.
10 "City of Medicine," The Encyclopedia of Greater Philadelphia, accessed November 4, 2024, https://philadelphiaencyclopedia.org/themes/city-of-medicine/#:~:text=For%20most%20of%20the%20nineteenth,as%20a%20city%20of%20medicine.
11 Thomas Pym Cope, *Passages From the Life and Writings of William Penn* (Philadelphia: For Sale At Friends' Book-Store, 1882), 263–64, HathiTrust.

12 "Poverty," The Encyclopedia of Greater Philadelphia, accessed October 10, 2024, https://philadelphiaencyclopedia.org/essays/poverty/.
13 Ibid.
14 Charles Lawrence, *History of the Philadelphia Almshouses and Hospitals* (self-pub., 1905), 19–20.
15 Thompson Westcott, *Historic Mansions and Buildings of Philadelphia* (Philadelphia: Porter & Coates, 1877), 98–99, HathiTrust.
16 *Minutes of the Common Council of the City of Philadelphia. 1704 to 1776* (Philadelphia: Crissy & Markley, 1847), 80, Internet Archive.
17 Gary B. Nash, "Poverty and Poor Relief in Pre-Revolutionary Philadelphia," *The William and Mary Quarterly* 33, no. 1 (Jan 1976): 5, JSTOR.
18 Lawrence, *History of the Philadelphia Almshouses and Hospitals*, 21.
19 Nash, "Poverty and Poor Relief in Pre-Revolutionary Philadelphia," 14.
20 Lawrence, *History of the Philadelphia Almshouses and Hospitals*, 22.
21 Simon, *Philadelphia: A Brief History*, 12.
22 Crist, "'The Mangled Remains of What Had Been Humanity': Evidence of Autopsy and Dissection at Philadelphia's Blockley Almshouse, 1835–1895," 262.
23 John K. Alexander, *Render Them Submissive: Responses to Poverty in Philadelphia, 1760–1800* (Amherst: The University of Massachusetts Press, 1980), 53.
24 Ibid., 6.
25 Benjamin Joseph Klebaner, "Employment of Paupers at Philadelphia's Almshouse Before 1861," *Pennsylvania History* 24, no. 2 (April 1957): 138, JSTOR; "Almshouse records Collection Am.3225," Historical Society of Pennsylvania, accessed October 28, 2024, https://www2.hsp.org/collections/manuscripts/a/AlmshouseAm3225.html.
26 "'Arator': On the Price of Corn, and Management of the Poor [29 November 1766]," Founders Online, accessed October 28, 2024, https://founders.archives.gov/documents/Franklin/01-13-02-0194.
27 Nash, "Poverty and Poor Relief in Pre-Revolutionary Philadelphia," 20.
28 Lawrence, *History of the Philadelphia Almshouses and Hospitals*, 66–67.
29 Billy G. Smith and Cynthia Shelton, "THE DAILY OCCURRENCE DOCKET OF THE PHILADELPHIA ALMSHOUSE: SELECTED ENTRIES, 1800–1804," *Pennsylvania History: A Journal of Mid-Atlantic Studies* 52, no. 3 (July 1985): 184, JSTOR.
30 Newman, *Embodied History: The Lives of the Poor in Early Philadelphia*, 22.
31 Lawrence, *History of the Philadelphia Almshouses and Hospitals*, 32.
32 Hunter, *The Origin of the Philadelphia General Hospital Blockley Division*, 13; Scharf and Westcott, *History of Philadelphia*, 2356; Lawrence, *History of the Philadelphia Almshouses and Hospitals*, 38.
33 Lawrence, *History of the Philadelphia Almshouses and Hospitals*, 33.
34 William Shippen Jr. to Thomas Lee Shippen, December 31, 1787, Shippen Family Papers, Library of Congress, Washington, D.C.

35 Lawrence, *History of the Philadelphia Almshouses and Hospitals*, 67–68.
36 Ibid., 68.
37 Ibid.
38 Isaac Ray, *What Shall Philadelphia Do for Its Paupers?* (Philadelphia: Social Science Association of Philadelphia, 1873), 2, National Library of Medicine.
39 Lawrence, *History of the Philadelphia Almshouses and Hospitals*, 57.
40 Ibid., 276.
41 Ibid., 320–22.
42 "Almshouses (Poorhouses)," The Encyclopedia of Greater Philadelphia, accessed October 30, 2024, https://philadelphiaencyclopedia.org/essays/almshouses-poorhouses/.
43 Simon, *Philadelphia: A Brief History*, 13.
44 Lawrence, *History of the Philadelphia Almshouses and Hospitals*, 85.
45 Newman, *Embodied History: The Lives of the Poor in Early Philadelphia*, 17.
46 Douglas Mooney and Kimberly Morrell, "Phase IB Archaeological Investigations of the Mother Bethel Burying Ground, Appendix A, Potter's Field and Almshouse Cemeteries in Philadelphia," accessed October 30, 2024, https://www.creativephl.org/wp-content/uploads/2020/12/Pt-Two-Appendix.pdf.
47 Ibid.
48 Robert J. Hunter, "The Origin of the Philadelphia General Hospital," *The Pennsylvania Magazine of History and Biography* 57, no. 1 (1933), 43, JSTOR; Hunter, *The Origin of the Philadelphia General Hospital Blockley Division*, 35.
49 Charles E. Rosenberg, "From Almshouse to Hospital: The Shaping of Philadelphia General Hospital," *The Milbank Memorial Fund Quarterly. Health and Society* 60, no. 1 (Winter 1982): 111, JSTOR.
50 William H. Williams, *America's First Hospital: The Pennsylvania Hospital, 1751–1841* (Pennsylvania: Haverford House, 1976), 7; Newman, *Embodied History*, 65.
51 Arthur Ames Bliss, *Blockley Days: Memories and Impressions of a Resident Physician 1883–1884* (Springfield Printing & Binding Co., 1916), 21–22.
52 Ibid.
53 Lawrence, *History of the Philadelphia Almshouses and Hospitals*, 339.
54 Ray, *What Shall Philadelphia Do for Its Paupers?*, 9.
55 Bliss, *Blockley Days*, 9.
56 Ibid., 68.
57 David Hayes Agnew, "The Medical History of the Philadelphia Almshouse," in *History of Blockley: A History of the Philadelphia General Hospital From Its Inception, 1731–1928*, ed. John Welsh Croskey (Philadelphia: F. A. Davis Company, 1929), 33.
58 Lawrence, *History of the Philadelphia Almshouses and Hospitals*, 35.
59 Ibid., 43.
60 Ibid.
61 William H. Williams, *America's First Hospital: The Pennsylvania Hospital, 1751–1841* (Pennsylvania: Haverford House, 1976), 139.

62 Lawrence, *History of the Philadelphia Almshouses and Hospitals*, 132.
63 Ibid., 105.
64 Agnew, *History and Reminiscences of the Philadelphia Almshouse and Philadelphia Hospital*, 22.
65 Sappol, *A Traffic of Dead Bodies*, 81.
66 John Harley Warner and James M. Edmonson, *Dissection: Photographs of a Rite of Passage in American Medicine 1880–1930* (New York: Blast Books, 2009), 7.
67 Leonard Warren, *Joseph Leidy: The Last Man Who Knew Everything* (New Haven: Yale University Press, 1998), 27.
68 Warner and Edmonson, *Dissection: Photographs of a Rite of Passage in American Medicine 1880–1930*, 9.
69 Bliss, *Blockley Days*, 24.
70 Lawrence, *History of the Philadelphia Almshouses and Hospitals*, 156.
71 Rosenberg, "From Almshouse to Hospital," 142.
72 Lawrence, *History of the Philadelphia Almshouses and Hospitals*, 58.
73 Rosenberg, "From Almshouse to Hospital," 110–11; Bliss, *Blockley Days*, 14.
74 Agnew, *History and Reminiscences of the Philadelphia Almshouse and Philadelphia Hospital*, 17.
75 Bliss, *Blockley Days*, 28, 30.
76 Ibid., 29.
77 Lawrence, *History of the Philadelphia Almshouses and Hospitals*, 160.
78 Ibid., 98, 255.
79 Ibid., 90.
80 J. Chalmers DaCosta, "The Old Blockley Hospital; Its Characters and Characteristics," *JAMA* L, no. 15 (April 11, 1908): 1183, JAMA.
81 Lawrence, *History of the Philadelphia Almshouses and Hospitals*, 160.
82 Ibid., 160.
83 Ibid., 160–61.
84 Ibid., 158.
85 Ibid., 253.
86 Guerrasio, "Dissecting the Pennsylvania Anatomy Act," 60.
87 Richardson, *Death, Dissection and the Destitute*, 128.
88 Lawrence, *History of the Philadelphia Almshouses and Hospitals*, 161.
89 Ibid., 162.
90 Douglas Mooney and Kimberly Morrell, "Phase IB Archaeological Investigations of the Mother Bethel Burying Ground, Appendix A, Potter's Field and Almshouse Cemeteries in Philadelphia," accessed October 30, 2024, https://www.creativephl.org/wp-content/uploads/2020/12/Pt-Two-Appendix.pdf.
91 DaCosta, "The Old Blockley Hospital; Its Characters and Characteristics," 1186.
92 Agnew, *History and Reminiscences of the Philadelphia Almshouse and Philadelphia Hospital*, 66.
93 Bliss, *Blockley Days*, 17.

94 Lawrence, *History of the Philadelphia Almshouses and Hospitals*, 156–57.
95 Bliss, *Blockley Days*, 89.
96 Lawrence, *History of the Philadelphia Almshouses and Hospitals*, 158.
97 Lawrence, *History of the Philadelphia Almshouses and Hospitals*, 158.
98 Ibid., 159.
99 Agnew, *History and Reminiscences of the Philadelphia Almshouse and Philadelphia Hospital*, 18.
100 Corner, *Two Centuries of Medicine*, 93.
101 Lawrence, *History of the Philadelphia Almshouses and Hospitals*, 208, 268.
102 Agnew, *History and Reminiscences of the Philadelphia Almshouse and the Philadelphia Hospital*, 97–98.
103 Lawrence, *History of the Philadelphia Almshouses and Hospitals*, 252.
104 Ibid., 264.
105 Ibid.
106 Edward Mussey Hartwell, "Hindrances to the Study of Anatomy," *The Medical and Surgical Reporter* VII, no. 25 (March 22, 1862): 596–97, Internet Archive.
107 Lawrence, *History of the Philadelphia Almshouses and Hospitals*, 270.
108 T. S. Sozinsky, "Grave-Robbing and Dissection," *The Penn Monthly* 10 (1879): 215, HathiTrust.
109 Lawrence, *History of the Philadelphia Almshouses and Hospitals*, 270.
110 "Subjects For Dissection," *The New York Times* (New York City, NY), Aug. 5, 1879, ProQuest.
111 "Anatomy and Anatomy Education," The Encyclopedia of Greater Philadelphia, accessed November 3, 2024, https://philadelphiaencyclopedia.org/essays/anatomy-and-anatomy-education/.
112 Agnew, *History and Reminiscences of the Philadelphia Almshouse and Philadelphia Hospital*, 33.
113 Bliss, *Blockley Days*, 17.
114 Agnew, *History and Reminiscences of the Philadelphia Almshouse and Philadelphia Hospital*, 134.
115 Carol Starr and William A. Gardner, "Philadelphia: Cradle of American Pathology," *Virchows Archiv* 458, no. 1 (2010), National Library of Medicine.
116 Kyla Downs & Paul Wolff Mitchell, "The Wistar Institute: From Anatomical Museum to Biomedical Research Center," accessed November 2, 2024, https://collaborativehistory.gse.upenn.edu/stories/wistar-institute-anatomical-museum-biomedical-research-center#fn06.
117 "Anatomy and Anatomy Education," The Encyclopedia of Greater Philadelphia.
118 Downs & Mitchell, "The Wistar Institute: From Anatomical Museum to Biomedical Research Center."
119 Sarah Laskow, "The Gruesome History of Making Human Skeletons," Atlas Obscura, last modified October 3, 2017, https://www.atlasobscura.com/articles/history-gruesome-skeleton-anatomists.

120 J. Howe Adams, *History of the Life of D. Hayes Agnew, M.D., LL.D.* (Philadelphia and London: The F. A. Davis Company, 1892), 71, Wellcome Collection.
121 Ibid., 71–72.
122 Paul Wolff Mitchell, "Black Philadelphians in the Samuel George Morton Cranial Collection," Penn Program On Race, Science & Society, last modified February 15, 2021, https://prss.sas.upenn.edu/projects/penn-medicines-role/black-philadelphians-samuel-george-morton-cranial-collection.
123 "The Complete Dissection of a Human Cerebrospinal Nervous System (Known as 'Harriet')," Drexel University Legacy Center Archives & Special Collections College of Medicine, accessed November 3, 2024, https://drexel.edu/legacy-center/the-collections/historical-human-remains/harrietcole-details/.
124 Jessica Leigh Hester, "The Mystery of 'Harriet Cole,'" Atlas Obscura, last modified March 18, 2021, https://www.atlasobscura.com/articles/harriet-cole-human-nervous-system-philadelphia.
125 "The Complete Dissection of a Human Cerebrospinal Nervous System (Known as 'Harriet')."
126 Hester, "The Mystery of 'Harriet Cole.'"
127 John Stockton Hough, "Two Cases of Trichiniasis observed at the Philadelphia Hospital, Blockley," *The American Journal of the Medical Sciences* 57, no. 114 (April 1869): 565, Ovid.
128 Megan Rosenbloom, *Dark Archives: A Librarian's Investigation Into the Science and History of Books Bound in Human Skin* (New York: Farrar, Straus and Giroux, 2020), 50.
129 "The Skin She Lived In: Anthropodermic Books in the Historical Medical Library," Fugitive Leaves, last modified October 1, 2025, https://histmed.collegeofphysicians.org/skin-she-lived-in/.
130 Ibid.
131 "Welcome to this inaugural edition of Fugitive Leaves…," Fugitive Leaves, last modified October 1, 2015, https://histmed.collegeofphysicians.org/welcome/.
132 Laura Ann Guelle, "Anthropodermic Book-Bindings," *Transactions & Studies of the College of Physicians of Philadelphia* XXIV, V (December 2002): 87, Internet Archive; Rosenbloom, *Dark Archives*, 56.
133 Jason Shwartz, "Classic texts—in the flesh," *The Daily Pennsylvanian*, January 18, 2006, https://www.thedp.com/article/2006/01/classic_texts_in_the_flesh; "The True Story of Medical Books Bound in Human Skin," Nautilus, last modified June 10, 2016, https://nautil.us/the-true-story-of-medical-books-bound-in-human-skin-235981/.
134 "The Anthropodermic Book Project," accessed November 7, 2024, https://anthropodermicbooks.org/.
135 Lawrence, *History of the Philadelphia Almshouses and Hospitals*, 306.
136 Donna Gentile O'Donnell, *Provider of Last Resort: The Story of the Philadelphia General Hospital* (Philadelphia: Camino Books, 2005), 9.

137 Ibid., 8.
138 "Philadelphia General Hospital (Old Blockley): Philadelphians 'Ain't Goin' to no Bellevue,'" PhilaPlace, accessed November 4, 2024, https://m.philaplace.org/story/897/.
139 Ibid.
140 Rosenberg, "From Almshouse to Hospital: The Shaping of Philadelphia General Hospital," 110; "Almshouse," Britannica, accessed November 3, 2024, https://www.britannica.com/topic/almshouse.
141 "Reburying the Past," *The Pennsylvania Gazette*, accessed November 6, 2024, https://thepenngazette.com/reburying-the-past/.
142 "The Philadelphia General Hospital: From Almshouse to Public Hospital and Beyond," West Philadelphia Collaborative History, accessed November 4, 2024, https://collaborativehistory.gse.upenn.edu/stories/philadelphia-general-hospital-almshouse-public-hospital-and-beyond.
143 Crist, "'The Mangled Remains of What Had Been Humanity': Evidence of Autopsy and Dissection at Philadelphia's Blockley Almshouse, 1835–1895," 264.
144 Ibid., 270.

Chapter 3: "The Philadelphia Method": Secret Agreements and the Cadaver Trade

1 William E. Horner to John Collins Warren, November 30, 1824, John Collins Warren Papers, Massachusetts Historical Society, quoted in Michael Sappol, *A Traffic of Dead Bodies: Anatomy and Embodied Social Identity in Nineteenth-Century America* (Princeton: Princeton University Press, 2002), 114.
2 "Excitement.—Dead Body Found," *Public Ledger* (Philadelphia, PA), October 13, 1846.
3 "Extinct Philadelphia Medical Schools," Penn Libraries, accessed July 30, 2024, https://archives.upenn.edu/exhibits/penn-history/medical-history/extinct/.
4 Baatz, "A Very Diffused Disposition," 213, JSTOR.
5 Sappol, *A Traffic of Dead Bodies*, 115.
6 James Webster, *Facts Concerning Anatomical Instruction in Philadelphia* (Philadelphia: 1832), 3, Wellcome Collection.
7 "Benjamin Franklin and the Pamphlet Wars," *Humanities: The Magazine of the National Endowment for the Humanities*, accessed August 1, 2024, https://www.neh.gov/article/benjamin-franklin-and-pamphlet-wars.
8 Webster, *Facts Concerning Anatomical Instruction in Philadelphia*, 7.
9 "The Late Dr. James Webster," *Boston Medical and Surgical Journal* 51, no. 11 (October 1854): 219; William W. Keen, *The History of the Philadelphia School of Anatomy and its Relations to Medical Teaching* (Philadelphia: J. B. Lippincott & Co., 1875), 11, Internet Archive.
10 Corner, *Two Centuries of Medicine*, 77.

11 James Webster, *Medical Intelligence* (Philadelphia: 1830), 3, Wellcome Collection.
12 Webster, *Facts Concerning Anatomical Instruction in Philadelphia*, 11.
13 Ibid.
14 Baatz, "A Very Diffused Disposition," 213.
15 Linden F. Edwards, "Dr. Frederick C. Waite's Correspondence With Reference to Grave Robbery," *The Ohio State Medical Journal* 54, no. 5 (1958): 602.
16 Webster, *Facts Concerning Anatomical Instruction in Philadelphia*, 5.
17 Ibid.
18 Ibid., 7.
19 Ibid., 7, 20.
20 James F. Gayley, *A History of The Jefferson Medical College of Philadelphia* (Philadelphia: Joseph M. Wilson, 1858), 16.
21 Keen, *The History of the Philadelphia School of Anatomy and its Relations to Medical Teaching*, 11.
22 Webster, *Facts Concerning Anatomical Instruction in Philadelphia*, 3.
23 Ibid., 6.
24 "The Late Dr. James Webster," *Boston Medical and Surgical Journal*, 219.
25 Sappol, *A Traffic of Dead Bodies*, 114.
26 John Davidson Godman to John Collins Warren, January 1, 1829, John Collins Warren Papers, Massachusetts Historical Society, quoted in Patsy Gerstner, "A Note on Body Snatching in the United States," *The Bulletin of the Cleveland Medical Library* 18, no. 7 (July 1971): 65.
27 Ibid.
28 Ibid.
29 Ibid.
30 Ibid.
31 William E. Horner to John Collins Warren, 30 November 1824, John Collins Warren Papers, Massachusetts Historical Society, quoted in Sappol, *A Traffic of Dead Bodies*, 114–15.
32 Sappol, *A Traffic of Dead Bodies*, 113, 125.
33 *Public Ledger* (Philadelphia, PA), September 26, 1841.
34 Laura Elizabeth Smith, "Dissection, Media Portrayals, and Reaction: Black Bodies and Medical Education in Nineteenth-Century Newspapers," *Clinical Anatomy* 37, no. 4 (February 2024): 459, Wiley.
35 "In Need of Cadavers, 19th-Century Medical Students Raided Baltimore's Graves," *Smithsonian Magazine*, October 25, 2018, https://www.smithsonianmag.com/history/in-need-cadavers-19th-century-medical-students-raided-baltimores-graves-180970629/.
36 "Arrest of Alleged Body Snatchers," *Evening Star* (Washington, D.C.), December 13, 1873, Library of Congress.
37 Frank Baker, "A History of Bodysnatching," in *Washington Medical Annals (Bimonthly) Journal of the Medical Society of the District of Columbia*, Vol. XV, 1916 (City of Washington: Beresford, Printer, 1916), 249, Internet Archive.

38 Ibid.
39 Ibid.
40 Thomas Dwight, *Anatomy Laws Versus Body-Snatching* (New York: Forum Pub. Co., 1896), 499.
41 Chester Dewey, *Introductory Lecture Delivered to the Medical Class of the Berkshire Medical Institution; August 5, 1847* (Pittsfield: Charles Montague, 1847), 25–26, quoted in Sappol, *A Traffic of Dead Bodies*, 122.
42 Waite, "Grave Robbing in New England," 283.
43 "Preservation of Bodies," *The Boston Medical and Surgical Journal* 13, no. 8 (September 30, 1835): 129, ProQuest.
44 Antero Pietila, *The Ghosts of Johns Hopkins: The Life and Legacy That Shaped an American City* (Lanham: Rowman & Littlefield, 2018), 79.
45 Keen, *The History of the Philadelphia School of Anatomy and its Relations to Medical Teaching*, 31.
46 Smith, "Dissection, Media Portrayals, and Reaction: Black Bodies and Medical Education in Nineteenth-Century Newspapers," 459.
47 Keen, *The History of the Philadelphia School of Anatomy and its Relations to Medical Teaching*, 8–9.
48 "The Resurrection Business," *Evening Star* (Washington, D.C.), December 15, 1873, 7, Library of Congress.
49 Ibid.
50 Baker, "A History of Bodysnatching," 251.
51 Ibid., 251.
52 Ibid., 249.
53 "A Student's Study," *Times-Picayune* (New Orleans, LA), November 7, 1878.
54 "Body Snatching in Ohio During the Nineteenth Century," *Ohio State Archaeological and Historical Quarterly*, 336, accessed November 1, 2024, https://resources.ohiohistory.org/ohj/search/display.php?page=76&ipp=20&searchterm=Array&vol=59&pages=329-351.
55 Linden F. Edwards, *Cincinnati's "Old Cunny": A Notorious Purveyor of Human Flesh* (Public Library of Fort Wayne and Allen County, 1955), 4, Project Gutenberg.
56 "'Stiff' Stealers: Grave Robbing in Atlanta," Historic Oakland Foundation, accessed August 22, 2024, https://oaklandcemetery.com/stiff-stealers/.
57 "Esprit De Corpse," *Washington City Paper*, accessed August 22, 2024, https://washingtoncitypaper.com/article/245113/esprit-de-corpse/.
58 Daniel Kilbride, "Southern Medical Students in Philadelphia, 1800–1861: Science and Sociability in the 'Republic of Medicine,'" *The Journal of Southern History* 65, no. 4 (November 1999): 705, JSTOR.
59 Lewis W. Minor to John S. Davis, November 30, 1850, Albert and Shirley Small Special Collections Library, University of Virginia.
60 Lewis W. Minor to John S. Davis, November 15, 1850, Albert and Shirley Small Special Collections Library, University of Virginia.

61 Breeden, "Body Snatchers and Anatomy Professors," 334.
62 Kirt von Daacke, "Anatomical Theater," in Maurie D. McInnis, Kirt von Daacke, Louis P. Nelson, and Benjamin Ford, eds., *Educated in Tyranny: Slavery at Thomas Jefferson's University* (Charlottesville: University of Virginia Press, 2019), 155, EBSCOhost.
63 E. F. Fontaine to John S. Davis, January 1, 1857, Albert and Shirley Small Special Collections Library, University of Virginia.
64 E. F. Fontaine to John S. Davis, October 24, 1851, Albert and Shirley Small Special Collections Library, University of Virginia.
65 John S. Davis to A. E. Peticolas, November 22, 1859, Albert and Shirley Small Special Collections Library, University of Virginia.
66 H. L. Thomas to John S. Davis, November 3, 1849, Albert and Shirley Small Special Collections Library, University of Virginia; John S. Davis to A. E. Peticolas, February 8, 1859, Albert and Shirley Small Special Collections Library, University of Virginia.
67 Edward C. Halperin, "The Poor, the Black, and the Marginalized as the Source of Cadavers in United States Anatomical Education," *Clinical Anatomy* 20, no. 5 (July 2007): 493, Wiley.
68 "Wholesale Body Snatching," *Galveston Daily News* (Galveston, TX), November 30, 1879.
69 "In Need of Cadavers, 19th-Century Medical Students Raided Baltimore's Graves," *Smithsonian Magazine*, accessed August 28, 2024, https://www.smithsonianmag.com/history/in-need-cadavers-19th-century-medical-students-raided-baltimores-graves-180970629/; Bruce Goldfarb, *OCME: Life in America's Top Forensic Medical Center* (Lebanon, New Hampshire: Steerforth, 2023), 21.
70 Daina Ramey Berry, *The Price for Their Pound of Flesh: The Value of the Enslaved, from Womb to Grave, in the Building of a Nation* (Boston: Beacon Press, 2017), 174.
71 "In Need of Cadavers, 19th-Century Medical Students Raided Baltimore's Graves," *Smithsonian Magazine*.
72 Oliver S. Hayward, "Three American Anatomy Letters (1817–1830)," *Bulletin of the History of Medicine* 38, no. 4 (July–August 1964): 378, JSTOR.
73 Stephen C. Kenny, "The Development of Medical Museums in the Antebellum American South: Slave Bodies in Networks of Anatomical Exchange," *Bulletin of the History of Medicine* 87, no. 1 (Spring 2013): 53, 56, JSTOR.
74 Daina Ramey Berry, "Beyond the Slave Trade, the Cadaver Trade," *The New York Times*, February 3, 2018, https://www.nytimes.com/2018/02/03/opinion/sunday/cadavers-slavery-medical-schools.html.
75 J. S. Buckingham, *America, Historical, Statistic, and Descriptive* (London: Fisher, Son & Co., 1841), Library of Congress, quoted in Walter Fisher, "Physicians and Slavery in the Antebellum Southern Medical Journal," *Journal of the History of Medicine and Allied Sciences* 23, no. 1 (January 1968): 45, JSTOR.
76 Harriet Martineau, *Retrospect of Western Travel Volume 1* (London: Saunders & Otley, 1838), 140, Library of Congress.

77 Waite, "Grave Robbing in New England," 284.
78 Gladys-Marie Fry, *Night Riders in Black Folk History* (Chapel Hill and London: The University of North Carolina Press, 1975), 171.
79 Smith, "Dissection, Media Portrayals, and Reaction: Black Bodies and Medical Education in Nineteenth-Century Newspapers," 464.
80 Fry, *Night Riders in Black Folk History*, 181.
81 "Medicine: Bodies by Bequest," *Time*, October 4, 1954, https://time.com/archive/6795030/medicine-bodies-by-bequest/.
82 Martin Kaufman and Leslie L. Hanawalt, "Body Snatching in the Midwest," *Michigan History Magazine* 55, no. 1 (1971): 39.
83 "Body Snatching in Ohio During the Nineteenth Century," *Ohio State Archaeological and Historical Quarterly,* 343–44, 346, accessed November 1, 2024, https://resources.ohiohistory.org/ohj/search/display.php?page=76&ipp=20&searchterm=Array&vol=59&pages=329-351.
84 "The Late Grave Robberies," *The Baltimore Sun* (Baltimore, MD), December 3, 1880, ProQuest.
85 "John Staige Davis (1824–1885)," Encyclopedia Virginia, accessed November 12, 2024, https://encyclopediavirginia.org/entries/davis-john-staige-1824-1885/.
86 John Y. Simon, *The Papers of Ulysses S. Grant, Volume 25: 1874* (Carbondale and Edwardsville: Southern Illinois University Press, 2003), 430.
87 "Dr. Christian, the Body-Snatcher," *Evening Star* (Washington, D.C.), June 11, 1878, 4, Library of Congress.
88 "Had Records As Ghouls," *The Times* (Washington, D.C.), February 24, 1896.
89 Baatz, "A Very Diffused Disposition," 212–13.
90 Ibid., 213.

Chapter 4: Body Snatching: Myth and Reality

1 Baker, "A History of Bodysnatching," 253.
2 "A Resurrectionist Punished," *Frank Leslie's Illustrated Newspaper* (New York City, NY), March 26, 1859, History Commons.
3 "The Body Snatchers—A Recent Actual Occurrence in the Vicinity of New York City," *Frank Leslie's Illustrated Newspaper* (New York City, NY), April 18, 1868, History Commons.
4 J. H. Robinson, *Marietta, Or The Two Students: A Tale of the Dissecting Room and "Body Snatchers"* (Boston: Jordan & Wiley, 1846), 10, Internet Archive.
5 Edwards, *Cincinnati's "Old Cunny,"* 1, Project Gutenberg.
6 Otto Juettner, *Daniel Drake and His Followers: Historical and Biographical Sketches* (Cincinnati: Harvey Publishing Company, 1909), 395, HathiTrust.
7 Ibid.
8 Edwards, *Cincinnati's "Old Cunny,"* 1.
9 Juettner, *Daniel Drake and His Followers*, 395.

10 Edwards, *Cincinnati's "Old Cunny,"* 4.
11 Ibid., 4.
12 Juettner, *Daniel Drake and His Followers*, 395.
13 Edwards, *Cincinnati's "Old Cunny,"* 8.
14 "Career of a Resurrectionist," *Chicago Daily Tribune* (Chicago, IL), November 7, 1887, ProQuest.
15 Baker, "A History of Bodysnatching," 251.
16 "Robbing the Graves of Their Dead," *The Washington Post* (Washington, D.C.), October 11, 1884, ProQuest.
17 "A King Among Ghouls," *The Washington Post* (Washington, D.C.), November 6, 1887, ProQuest.
18 "Career of a Resurrectionist," *Chicago Daily Tribune* (Chicago, IL), November 7, 1887, ProQuest.
19 "A King Among Ghouls," *The Washington Post.*
20 "Had Records As Ghouls," *The Times* (Washington, D.C.), February 24, 1896.
21 Ibid.
22 "Vigo Jansen: The Resurrectionist King," Boundary Stones: WETA'S Local History Website, last updated October 30, 2015, https://boundarystones.weta.org/2015/10/30/vigo-jansen-resurrectionist-king#footnote-2.
23 "The Resurrectionist King," *The Washington Post* (Washington, D.C.), May 19, 1884, ProQuest.
24 "Vigo Jansen: The Resurrectionist King," Boundary Stones: WETA'S Local History Website.
25 "A King Among Ghouls," *The Washington Post.*
26 "The Theft of Corpses," *The Washington Post* (Washington, D.C.), December 29, 1889, ProQuest.
27 "A King Among Ghouls," *The Washington Post.*
28 Edward Warren, *The Life of John Collins Warren, M.D. Compiled Chiefly From His Autobiography and Journals in Two Volumes. Vol. I* (Boston: Ticknor and Fields, 1860), 404, Google Books.
29 Edward H. Dixon, "Scenes in a Medical Student's Life—Resurrectionizing," *Scalpel: An Entirely Original Quarterly Expositor of the Laws of Health, and Abuses of Medicine and Domestic Life* 7 (1855): 93, Gale.
30 Ibid., 96.
31 "Resurrectionists' Methods," *The New York Times* (New York City, NY), August 16, 1878, ProQuest.
32 Kaufman and Hanawalt, "Body Snatching in the Midwest," 31–32.
33 Howard A. Kelly and Walter L. Burrage, *American Medical Biographies* (Baltimore: The Norman, Remington Company, 1920), 471, Wikisource.
34 Arthur M. Lassek, *Human Dissection: Its Drama and Struggle* (Springfield, Illinois: Charles C. Thomas, 1958), 222, Internet Archive.
35 Ibid.

36 Kelly and Burrage, *American Medical Biographies*, 471.
37 Juettner, *Daniel Drake and His Followers*, 392, HathiTrust.
38 A. E. Peticolas to John S. Davis, January 21, 1856, Albert and Shirley Small Special Collections Library, University of Virginia.
39 Richardson, *Death, Dissection and the Destitute*, 70.
40 Baker, "A History of Bodysnatching," 247.
41 Kaufman and Hanawalt, "Body Snatching in the Midwest," 31–37.
42 Dixon, "Scenes in a Medical Student's Life—Resurrectionizing," 94.
43 "Confessions of a Body-Snatcher," *The New York Times* (New York City, NY), November 18, 1878, ProQuest.
44 Cal Samra, "U-M No Longer Has To Buy—or Steal—Cadavers," *Ann Arbor News* (Ann Arbor, MI), October 24, 1971, Ann Arbor District Library.
45 Waite, "Grave Robbing in New England," 280.
46 Ibid.
47 "The Resurrection Business," *Evening Star* (Washington, D.C.), December 15, 1873, 7, Library of Congress.
48 Berry, *The Price for Their Pound of Flesh*, 165.
49 Suzie Lennox, *Bodysnatchers: Digging Up the Untold Stories of Britain's Resurrection Men* (Great Britain: Pen & Sword History, 2016), 56.
50 "The College Horror," *The Cincinnati Daily Enquirer* (Cincinnati, OH), June 4, 1878, ProQuest.
51 "The Resurrection Business," *Evening Star* (Washington, D.C.), December 15, 1873, 7, Library of Congress.
52 Baker, "A History of Bodysnatching," 251.
53 Henry Lonsdale, *A Sketch of the Life and Writings of Robert Knox The Anatomist* (London: Macmillan and Co., 1870), 103–4, Internet Archive, quoted in Shultz, *Body Snatching: The Robbing of Graves for the Education of Physicians in Early Nineteenth Century America*, 26–27.
54 Ibid., 104–5.
55 H. L. Thomas to J. S. Davis, August 31, 1849, Albert and Shirley Small Special Collections Library, University of Virginia.
56 Shultz, *Body Snatching: The Robbing of Graves for the Education of Physicians in Early Nineteenth Century America*, 35.
57 Bailey, *The Diary of a Resurrectionist 1811–1812*, 124.
58 George MacGregor, *The History of Burke and Hare and of the Resurrectionist Times: A Fragment From the Criminal Annals of Scotland* (Glasgow: Thomas D. Morison, 1884), 64, Internet Archive.
59 Bailey, *The Diary of a Resurrectionist 1811–1812*, 149, 155.
60 Breeden, "Body Snatchers and Anatomy Professors," 332.
61 Richardson, *Death, Dissection and the Destitute*, 59.
62 Shultz, *Body Snatching: The Robbing of Graves for the Education of Physicians in Early Nineteenth Century America*, 35.

63 "Thomas Wakley, The Founder of 'The Lancet.' A Biography," *The Lancet* 147, no. 3777 (January 18, 1896): 187, quoted in Shultz, *Body Snatching: The Robbing of Graves for the Education of Physicians in Early Nineteenth Century America*, 34.
64 Waite, "Grave Robbing in New England," 280.
65 Dixon, "Scenes in a Medical Student's Life—Resurrectionizing," 95.
66 Warren, *The Life of John Collins Warren, M.D. Compiled Chiefly From His Autobiography and Journals in Two Volumes. Vol. I*, 404.
67 Ibid., 405.
68 Bransby Blake Cooper, *The Life of Sir Astley Cooper, Vol. 1* (London: John W. Parker, West Strand, 1843), 353, Google Books.
69 Richardson, *Death, Dissection and the Destitute*, 59.
70 Juettner, *Daniel Drake and His Followers: Historical and Biographical Sketches*, 394.
71 Richardson, *Death, Dissection and the Destitute*, 59.
72 Cooper, *The Life of Sir Astley Cooper, Vol. 1*, 355.
73 "Resurrectionists' Methods," *The New York Times* (New York City, NY), August 16, 1878, ProQuest.
74 "Raising the Dead," *The Washington Post* (Washington, D.C.), April 1, 1883, 7, ProQuest.
75 "About Resurrectionists," *The New Bloomfield Times* (New Bloomfield, PA), April 20, 1880, 3, Newspapers.com.
76 "Arrest of the Alleged Body Snatchers," *Evening Star* (Washington, D.C.), December 13, 1873, 8, Library of Congress.
77 Waite, "Grave Robbing in New England," 280.
78 "Confession of Ghouls," *The Indianapolis Journal* (Indianapolis, IN), September 30, 1902, 1, 7, Library of Congress.
79 "Cantrell, The Philadelphia Grave-Robber," *The World's News* (Sydney, AU), April 11, 1903.
80 "The Resurrectionists," *Frank Leslie's Illustrated Newspaper* (New York City, NY), January 6, 1866, History Commons.
81 William Holtz, "Bankrobbers, Burkers, and Bodysnatchers," *Michigan Quarterly Review* 6, no. 2 (1967): 91.
82 Lewis W. Minor to John Staige Davis September 19, 1850, Albert and Shirley Small Special Collections Library, University of Virginia.
83 Janne Sager, "Most Americans Are Too Fat to Donate their Bodies to Science," Vice, accessed November 1, 2024, https://www.vice.com/en/article/most-americans-are-too-fat-to-donate-their-bodies-to-science/#:~:text=As%20in%2C%20the%20average%20American,or%20longer%20than%206%E2%80%B2%20tall.
84 "FAQ," Humanity Gifts Registry, accessed December 1, 2024, http://www.hgrpa.org/faq.
85 "The Body Snatchers—A Recent Actual Occurrence in the Vicinity of New York City," *Frank Leslie's Illustrated Newspaper* (New York City, NY), April 18, 1868, History Commons.

86 "The Resurrectionists," *Frank Leslie's Illustrated Newspaper* (New York City, NY), January 6, 1866, History Commons.
87 H. L. Thomas to J. S. Davis September 5, 1849, Albert and Shirley Small Special Collections Library, University of Virginia.
88 "The Resurrection Business," *Evening Star* (Washington, D.C.), December 15, 1873, 7, Library of Congress.
89 Killis Campbell, *The Mind of Poe and Other Studies* (Cambridge, Massachusetts: Harvard University Press, 1933), 167.
90 Bailey, *The Diary of a Resurrectionist 1811–1812*, 174.
91 "George Washington's Dentures FAQ," George Washington's Mount Vernon, accessed September 15, 2024, https://www.mountvernon.org/george-washington/health/washingtons-teeth/teeth/.
92 "The Trouble with Teeth," George Washington's Mount Vernon, accessed September 15, 2024, https://www.mountvernon.org/george-washington/health/washingtons-teeth/.
93 Eric Grundhauser, "When Dentures Used Real Human Teeth," Atlas Obscura, accessed September 15, 2024, https://www.atlasobscura.com/articles/when-dentures-used-real-human-teeth#:~:text=But%20in%20the%20dark%20ages,good%20teeth%20from%20battlefield%20casualties.
94 MacGregor, *The History of Burke and Hare and of the Resurrectionist Times*, 100.
95 Ibid.
96 *Philadelphia Repertory* 1, no. 26 (October 27, 1810): 207, EBSCOhost.
97 "The Avondale Murder," *The Cincinnati Enquirer* (Cincinnati, OH), May 1, 1884, Newspapers.com.
98 "Body Snatching in Ohio During the Nineteenth Century," *Ohio State Archaeological and Historical Quarterly*, 350, accessed November 1, 2024, https://resources.ohiohistory.org/ohj/search/display.php?page=76&ipp=20&searchterm=Array&vol=59&pages=329-351.
99 "Robbing the Hangman," *The Cincinnati Enquirer* (Cincinnati, OH), May 1, 1884, Newspapers.com.
100 Richard O Jones, "The Avondale Horror: Cincinnati's 1884 Burking Murders," accessed November 1, 2024, https://beltmag.com/avondale-horror-cincinnatis-1884-burking-murders/.
101 "Execution of Ross," *The Sun* (Baltimore, MD), September 10, 1887, ProQuest.
102 Ibid.
103 Ibid.
104 Robert Louis Stevenson, *Tales and Fantasies*, accessed November 19, 2024 https://www.gutenberg.org/files/426/426-h/426-h.htm.
105 Ibid.
106 Ibid.
107 Ibid.
108 "Edgar Allan Poe National Historic Site Pennsylvania," National Park Service, accessed November 17, 2024, https://www.nps.gov/edal/index.htm.

109 Ann K. Johnson, "Book Publishing and Publishers," accessed November 17, 2024, https://philadelphiaencyclopedia.org/essays/book-publishing-and-publishers/.
110 Edgar Allan Poe, "The Fall of the House of Usher," Project Gutenberg, accessed November 17, 2024, https://www.gutenberg.org/cache/epub/932/pg932-images.html.
111 "Quaker City (The); Or, the Monks of Monk Hall," The Encyclopedia of Greater Philadelphia, accessed November 23, 2024, https://philadelphiaencyclopedia.org/essays/quaker-city-novel/.
112 Ibid.
113 George Lippard, *The Quaker City; or, The Monks of Monk Hall: A Romance of Philadelphia Life, Mystery, and Crime* (Philadelphia: Leary, Stuart & Company, 1845), 91, Internet Archive.
114 Ibid.
115 Ibid.
116 "Edgar Allen Poe House," ushistory.org, accessed November 24, 2024, https://www.ushistory.org/tour/edgar-allan-poe-house.htm.
117 Baker, "A History of Bodysnatching," 247.

Chapter 5: Defending the Dead: Cemetery Guns, Coffin Torpedoes, and Cremation

1 "Victorian 'Coffin Torpedoes' Blasted Would-Be Body Snatchers," Atlas Obscura, accessed April 28, 2024, https://www.atlasobscura.com/articles/coffin-torpedos.
2 "1017 VERY RARE ASH STEEL AND WROUGHT-IRON CEMETERY GUN, ENGLAND, 18TH/EARLY 19TH CENTURY," Sotheby's, accessed April 28, 2024, https://www.sothebys.com/en/auctions/ecatalogue/2016/schorsch-collection-n09466/lot.1017.html.
3 "The Resurrectionists," *Frank Leslie's Weekly* (New York City, NY), January 6, 1866, History Commons.
4 "The 'Cemetery Gun': One Defense Against Grave Robbers," Slate, accessed April 28, 2024, https://slate.com/human-interest/2013/01/cemetery-gun-invented-to-thwart-grave-robbers.html.
5 "1017 VERY RARE ASH STEEL AND WROUGHT-IRON CEMETERY GUN, ENGLAND, 18TH/EARLY 19TH CENTURY," Sotheby's.
6 "Victorian 'Coffin Torpedoes' Blasted Would-Be Body Snatchers."
7 Sherry Carpenter, "Group Dispels Myth About Covered Plot," *The Daily Item* (Sunbury, PA), October 31, 2004, Newspapers.com.
8 Chris Krepich, "Historians Restore Franklin Landmark," *Press Enterprise* (Bloomsburg, PA), November 14, 1999, Newspapers.com.
9 Ann F. Diseroad, "Were they to keep the dead in…or the living out? CAGES ON GRAVES EXPLAINED A Wee Bit of Olde Scotland Right Here in Columbia County," Columbia County Historical & Genealogical Society Newsletter Article,

accessed April 27, 2024, https://colcohist-gensoc.org/wp-content/uploads/Cages%20on%20Graves%20Explained.pdf.

10 Allison C. Meier, "Beating the Bodysnatchers," Wellcome Collection, June 14, 2018, https://wellcomecollection.org/stories/beating-the-bodysnatchers.

11 James Ritchie, "RELICS OF THE BODY-SNATCHERS: SUPPLEMENTARY NOTES ON MORTSAFE TACKLE, MORTSAFES, WATCH-HOUSES, AND PUBLIC VAULTS, MOSTLY IN ABERDEENSHIRE," *Proceedings of the Society of Antiquaries of Scotland* (March 14, 1921): 221.

12 Ritchie, "RELICS OF THE BODY-SNATCHERS: SUPPLEMENTARY NOTES ON MORTSAFE TACKLE, MORTSAFES, WATCH-HOUSES, AND PUBLIC VAULTS, MOSTLY IN ABERDEENSHIRE."

13 Diseroad, "CAGES ON GRAVES EXPLAINED," 2.

14 "Hooded Graves Near Catawissa," *The Morning Press* (Bloomsburg, PA), August 9, 1963; ibid., 2–3.

15 Chris Krepich, "Historians Restore Franklin Landmark," *Press Enterprise* (Bloomsburg, PA), November 14, 1999, Newspapers.com; Diseroad, "CAGES ON GRAVES EXPLAINED," 2.

16 Bransby Blake Cooper, *The Life of Sir Astley Cooper, Vol. 1* (London: John W. Parker, West Strand, 1843), 352, Google Books.

17 Ibid.

18 James Ritchie, "AN ACCOUNT OF THE WATCH-HOUSES, MORTSAFES, AND PUBLIC VAULTS IN ABERDEENSHIRE CHURCHYARDS, FORMERLY USED FOR THE PROTECTION OF THE DEAD FROM THE RESURRECTIONISTS," *Proceedings of the Society of Antiquaries of Scotland* (March 11, 1912): 298.

19 Ibid., 295.

20 Waite, "Grave Robbing in New England," 277.

21 "An Easy Way To Secure Dead Bodies In Their Graves," *Freedom's Journal* (New York City, NY), March 30, 1827.

22 "Woodlands Cemetery," Historic American Landscapes Survey, accessed April 29, 2024, https://memory.loc.gov/master/pnp/habshaer/pa/pa4000/pa4013/data/pa4013data.pdf, 40.

23 Todd Harra, *Last Rites: The Evolution of the American Funeral* (Boulder, Colorado: Sounds True, 2022), 134.

24 "WATCHING THE GRAVES. HOW PHILADELPHIA CEMETERIES ARE PROTECTED," *The New York Times* (New York City, NY), December 3, 1878, ProQuest.

25 "The Resurrection Business," *Evening Star* (Washington, D.C.), December 15, 1873, Library of Congress.

26 "WATCHING THE GRAVES. HOW PHILADELPHIA CEMETERIES ARE PROTECTED," *New York Times*.

27 Baker, "A History of Bodysnatching," 248.

28 Ibid., 249.

29 "WATCHING THE GRAVES. HOW PHILADELPHIA CEMETERIES ARE PROTECTED," *New York Times*.
30 Ibid.
31 Ibid.
32 Ritchie, "AN ACCOUNT OF THE WATCH-HOUSES, MORTSAFES, AND PUBLIC VAULTS IN ABERDEENSHIRE CHURCHYARDS, FORMERLY USED FOR THE PROTECTION OF THE DEAD FROM THE RESURRECTIONISTS," 289.
33 "A New Form of Madness," *The Times* (Philadelphia, PA), March 29, 1883.
34 "The Resurrectionists," *Frank Leslie's Weekly*.
35 Dr. Frederick C. Waite, "Dr. Frederick C. Waite's Correspondence With Reference to Grave Robbery," *The Ohio State Medical Journal* 54, no. 5 (1958): 602.
36 "A Grave Robber Shot Dead," *New York Times* (New York City, NY), February 26, 1897.
37 Ritchie, "AN ACCOUNT OF THE WATCH-HOUSES, MORTSAFES, AND PUBLIC VAULTS IN ABERDEENSHIRE CHURCHYARDS, FORMERLY USED FOR THE PROTECTION OF THE DEAD FROM THE RESURRECTIONISTS," 289.
38 "Nervous Grave Guards," *The Times* (Philadelphia, PA), December 8, 1884.
39 Warren, *The Life of John Collins Warren, M.D. Compiled Chiefly From His Autobiography and Journals in Two Volumes. Vol. I*, 408.
40 "A Horror," *Cincinnati Commercial Tribune* (Cincinnati, OH), May 31, 1878.
41 Ibid.
42 Ibid.
43 Ibid.
44 "Human Hyenas," *Cincinnati Enquirer* (Cincinnati, OH), May 31, 1878.
45 Ibid.
46 Ibid.
47 "A Horror," *Cincinnati Commercial Tribune*, May 31, 1878.
48 Ibid.
49 Harry J. Sievers, *The Harrison Horror* (Fort Wayne: Public Library of Fort Wayne and Allen County, 1956), 38, HathiTrust.
50 Linden F. Edwards, "The Famous Harrison Case and Its Repercussions," *Bulletin of the History of Medicine* 31, no. 2 (March–April 1957): 165, JSTOR.
51 Sievers, *The Harrison Horror*, 30.
52 Ibid., 33.
53 "A Torpedo Blows Them Up," *The Stark County Democrat* (Canton, OH), January 20, 1881, Library of Congress.
54 Philip K. Clover. 1878. Improvement in Coffin-Torpedoes. US Patent 208,672, filed June 29, 1878, and issued October 8, 1878.
55 Ibid.; "Burial Devices," *New-York Tribune* (New York City, NY), August 14, 1896, ProQuest.

56 Philip K. Clover. 1878. Improvement in Coffin-Torpedoes. US Patent 208,672, filed June 29, 1878, and issued October 8, 1878.
57 T. N. Howell. Grave-Torpedo. US Patent 217,379, filed May 8, 1879, and issued July 8, 1879.
58 Ibid.
59 "The Torpedo of the Grave," *Norfolk Virginian* (Norfolk, VA), December 6, 1878.
60 T. N. Howell. Grave-Torpedo. US Patent 251,231, October 24, 1881, and issued December 20, 1881.
61 "Bombs Guard Her Grave," *The Topeka State Journal* (Topeka, KS), May 15, 1899, Library of Congress, quoted in Lucy Tiven, "Victorian 'Coffin Torpedoes' Blasted Would-Be Body Snatchers," Atlas Obscura, accessed November 1, 2024, https://www.atlasobscura.com/articles/coffin-torpedos.
62 Thomas J. Craughwell, *Stealing Lincoln's Body* (Cambridge, Massachusetts: The Belknap Press of Harvard University Press, 2007), 102.
63 Peggy Robertson, "The Plot to Steal Lincoln's Body," *American Heritage* 33, no. 3 (April/May 1982), https://www.americanheritage.com/plot-steal-lincolns-body.
64 Ibid.
65 Craughwell, *Stealing Lincoln's Body*, 175, 194–95.
66 Harra, *Last Rites: The Evolution of the American Funeral*, 133.
67 Andrew Van Bibber. Improvement in Burial-Safes. US Patent 207,570, filed August 5, 1878, and issued August 27, 1878.
68 Harra, *Last Rites: The Evolution of the American Funeral*, 139.
69 Andrew Van Bibber. Improvement in Burial-Safes. US Patent 207,570, filed August 5, 1878, and issued August 27, 1878.
70 George W. Boyd. Burial-Case. US Patent 220,119, filed February 5, 1879, and issued September 30, 1879.
71 *Bloomington Evening World* (Bloomington, IN), August 19, 1901.
72 "Guarding Against Grave-Robbers," *The New York Times* (New York City, NY), December 27, 1881, ProQuest.
73 James Shannon. Improvement in Coffins. US Patent 212,273, filed December 11, 1878, and issued February 11, 1879.
74 Lucy Tiven, "Victorian 'Coffin Torpedoes' Blasted Would-Be Body Snatchers," Atlas Obscura, accessed November 1, 2024, https://www.atlasobscura.com/articles/coffin-torpedos.
75 "Precautions in Philadelphia Cemeteries," *The Jeffersonian-Democrat* (Brookville, PA), December 11, 1878, Newspapers.com.
76 "Burial Devices," *New-York Tribune* (New York City, NY), August 14, 1896, ProQuest.
77 William E. Horner, *Necrological Notice of Dr. Philip Syng Physick* (Philadelphia: Haswell, Barrington, and Haswell, 1838), 17–18, Internet Archive.
78 Thomas N. Haviland, "Benjamin Rush, Philip Syng Physick, and the Resurrectionists," *Surgery, Gynecology & Obstetrics* 117 (1963): 775.
79 Ibid., 774.

80 Thomas W. Laqueur, *The Work of the Dead: A Cultural History of Mortal Remains* (Princeton and Oxford: Princeton University Press, 2015), 1, 3.
81 T. S. Sozinsky, "Grave Robbing and Dissection," *Penn Monthly* 10 (1879): 208, HathiTrust.
82 "Grave Robbing," *The Philadelphia Inquirer* (Philadelphia, PA), June 28, 1878, ProQuest.
83 Robert Southey, *Poems* (1799), Project Gutenberg, https://www.gutenberg.org/files/8639/8639-h/8639-h.htm#section13.
84 Edward Warren, *The Life of John Collins Warren, M.D. Compiled Chiefly from His Autobiography and Journals in Two Volumes, Vol. II* (Boston: Ticknor and Fields, 1860), 359, Google Books.
85 Stephen Prothero, *Purified by Fire: A History of Cremation in America* (Berkeley: University of California Press, 2001), 58.
86 Ibid., 6.
87 Ibid., 214.
88 "Cremating the Dead," *The Philadelphia Inquirer* (Philadelphia, PA), December 7, 1882.
89 "Grave Robberies and Cremation," *The Philadelphia Inquirer* (Philadelphia, PA), August 12, 1891.
90 "Graves Robbed and Desecrated," *The Urn* (New York City, NY), September 25, 1895, ProQuest; "Cremation In Its Sanitary Aspects," *The Urn* (New York City, NY), March 25, 1894, ProQuest.
91 Hugo Erichsen, *The Cremation of the Dead* (Detroit: D. O. Haynes & Company, 1887), 154, Internet Archive.
92 Prothero, *Purified by Fire*, 26.
93 "II, 14 December 1799," Founders Online, accessed December 7, 2024, https://founders.archives.gov/documents/Washington/06-04-02-0406-0002.
94 "Keeps Husband's Body 2 Weeks After Death," *The Washington Herald* (Washington, D.C), October 5, 1913, Library of Congress.
95 Ibid.
96 Henry H. Windsor, "Odd Family Vault Prevents Premature Burial," *Popular Mechanics* 36 (July 1921).
97 Samuel D. Gross, *Autobiography of Samuel D. Gross, M.D. Vol. II* (Philadelphia: George Barrie, Publisher, 1887), 210, Google Books.
98 "Ohio's Ghoulish Gambit Against Grave Robbing: Coffin Torpedoes," WOSU Public Media, accessed November 1, 2024, https://www.wosu.org/news/2017-05-17/ohios-ghoulish-gambit-against-grave-robbing-coffin-torpedoes.

Chapter 6: "A Resurrectionist Punished": Body Snatching and the Law

1 "The British Medical Association Meeting at Toronto," *The Lancet* 168, no. 4332 (September 8, 1906): 672, Elsevier.

2 W. J. McKnight, *A Pioneer Outline History of Northwestern Pennsylvania* (Philadelphia: J. B. Lippincott Company, 1905), 288.
3 "Medicine (Colonial Era)," The Encyclopedia of Greater Philadelphia, accessed December 15, 2024, https://philadelphiaencyclopedia.org/essays/medicine-colonial-era/.
4 McKnight, *A Pioneer Outline History of Northwestern Pennsylvania*, 289.
5 Ibid., 293.
6 W. J. McKnight, *A Pioneer History of Jefferson County, Pennsylvania* (Philadelphia: J. B. Lippincott Company, 1898), 556, Library of Congress.
7 McKnight, *A Pioneer Outline History of Northwestern Pennsylvania*, 294.
8 Ibid.
9 Ibid.
10 Ibid., 296.
11 Ibid., 291.
12 Ibid., 293.
13 Sappol, *A Traffic of Dead Bodies*, 101.
14 Baker, "A History of Bodysnatching," 249.
15 "Had Records as Ghouls," *The Times* (Washington, D.C.), February 24, 1896, Newspapers.com.
16 "Dissection Riots," *The Philadelphia Press* (Philadelphia, PA), December 11, 1882.
17 "A Ghastly Discovery," *The New York Times* (New York City, NY), December 23, 1887, ProQuest.
18 "Pickled," *Cincinnati Enquirer* (Cincinnati, OH), August 6, 1878, ProQuest.
19 "Dissection Riots," *The Philadelphia Press* (Philadelphia, PA), December 11, 1882.
20 "Pillory," Britannica, accessed December 22, 2024, https://www.britannica.com/topic/pillory-penology.
21 Wilf, "Anatomy and Punishment in Late Eighteenth-Century New York," 514.
22 Waite, "Grave Robbing in New England," 274.
23 Sappol, *A Traffic of Dead Bodies*, 102.
24 Rachel H. Mathis, Jill H. Watras, Jonathan M. Dort, "Grave Robbing in the North and South in Antebellum America," American College of Surgeons, 2016, 17, https://www.facs.org/media/1x0f0byz/03_grave_robbing.pdf.
25 Ibid.
26 Frederick C. Waite, "The Development of Anatomical Laws in the States of New England," *The New England Journal of Medicine* 233, no. 24 (December 13, 1945): 721.
27 Linden F. Edwards, "The Ohio Anatomy Law of 1881," *The Ohio State Medical Journal* 47, no. 2 (1951): 144.
28 *Laws of the General Assembly of the Commonwealth of Pennsylvania, Passed At the Session of 1849, in the Seventy-Third Year of Independence, with an Appendix* (Harrisburg, PA: J. M. G. Lescure, 1849), 397, Google Books.
29 *Laws of the General Assembly of the Commonwealth of Pennsylvania, Passed At the Session of 1855, in the Seventy-Ninth Year of Independence, with an Appendix* (Harrisburg, PA: A. Boyd Hamilton, 1855), 463, Google Books.

30 Warren, *The Life of John Collins Warren, M.D. Compiled Chiefly From His Autobiography and Journals in Two Volumes. Vol. I*, 406, Google Books.
31 Moore, *The Knife Man*, 40.
32 Sievers, *The Harrison Horror*, 11.
33 "A Robber of Graves," *The New York Times* (New York City, NY), January 31, 1878, ProQuest.
34 Edwards, *Cincinnati's "Old Cunny,"* 3, Project Gutenberg.
35 Ibid., 2.
36 Bess Lovejoy, "Meet Grandison Harris, the Grave Robber Enslaved (and then Employed) By the Georgia Medical College," *Smithsonian Magazine*, accessed December 2, 2024, https://www.smithsonianmag.com/history/meet-grandison-harris-grave-robber-enslaved-and-then-employed-georgia-college-medicine-180951344/.
37 Berry, *The Price for Their Pound of Flesh*, 170.
38 Daina Ramey Berry, "Beyond the Slave Trade, the Cadaver Trade," *The New York Times* (New York City, NY), February 3, 2018, https://www.nytimes.com/2018/02/03/opinion/sunday/cadavers-slavery-medical-schools.html.
39 Kirt von Daacke, "Anatomical Theater," in Maurie D. McInnis, Kirt von Daacke, Louis P. Nelson, and Benjamin Ford, eds., *Educated in Tyranny: Slavery at Thomas Jefferson's University* (Charlottesville: University of Virginia Press, 2019), 143, EBSCOhost.
40 "A Resurrectionist Punished," *Frank Leslie's Illustrated Newspaper* (New York City, NY), March 26, 1859, History Commons.
41 Ibid.
42 Edward B. Krumbhaar, "The Early History of Anatomy in the United States," *Annals of Medical History* 4, no. 3 (September 1922): 284, PubMed.
43 Hannibal Hamlin, "The Dissection Riot of 1824 and the Connecticut Anatomy Law," *Yale Journal of Biology and Medicine* 7, no. 4 (March 1935): 284.
44 John McNab Currier, *Song of Hubbardton Raid* (Castleton, Vermont, 1880), Wikisource, https://en.wikisource.org/wiki/Song_of_Hubbardton_Raid.
45 Ibid.
46 James Walter Wilson, "Joseph Nash McDowell, M.D.," *The Register of the Kentucky Historical Society* 68, no. 4 (October 1970): 343, JSTOR.
47 Luke Ritter, "Anatomy, Grave-Robbing, and Spiritualism in Antebellum St. Louis," *The Confluence* (Spring/Summer 2012): 36.
48 Juettner, *Daniel Drake and His Followers*, 393.
49 Waite, "Grave Robbing in New England," 285.
50 Baker, "A History of Bodysnatching," 248.
51 "Body Snatching in Ohio During the Nineteenth Century," *Ohio State Archaeological and Historical Quarterly*, 344, *https://resources.ohiohistory.org/ohj/search/display.php?page=76&ipp=20&searchterm=Array&vol=59&pages=329-351.*
52 John B. Blake, "The Development of American Anatomy Acts," *Journal of Medical Education* 30, no. 8 (August 1955): 434, Ovid.

53 William W. Keen, *The History of the Philadelphia School of Anatomy and its Relations to Medical Teaching* (Philadelphia: J. B. Lippincott & Co., 1875), 31, Internet Archive.
54 William Holtz, "Bankrobbers, Burkers, and Bodysnatchers," *Michigan Quarterly Review* 6, no. 2 (1967): 92.
55 Baker, "A History of Bodysnatching," 248.
56 Charles Goodall, *The Royal College of Physicians of London* (London: Bishop's Head, 1684), 24, Internet Archive.
57 *The Colonial Laws of Massachusetts* (Boston: F. B. Rothman & Co., 1889), 43, Internet Archive.
58 *Acts and Resolves of Massachusetts. 1784–85* (Boston: Adams & Nourse, n.d.), 25, Internet Archive.
59 Sappol, *A Traffic of Dead Bodies*, 109.
60 Wilf, "Anatomy and Punishment in Late Eighteenth-Century New York," 507, 514, 523.
61 Walter Hellerstein, "'Body-Snatching' Reconsidered: The Exhumation of Some Early American Legal History," *Brooklyn Law Review* 39, no. 2 (Summer 1972), 363–64, Digital Commons.
62 Wilf, "Anatomy and Punishment in Late Eighteenth-Century New York," 516.
63 Hamlin, "The Dissection Riot of 1824 and the Connecticut Anatomical Law," 286.
64 Thomas Francis Harrington, *The Harvard Medical School: A History, Narrative and Documentary* (New York: Lewis Publishing Company, 1905), 661, Google Books.
65 Waite, "The Development of Anatomical Laws in the States of New England," 721.
66 "Thomas Wakley, The Founder of 'The Lancet.' A Biography," *The Lancet* 147, no. 3777 (January 18, 1896): 187.
67 John Bishop, *A Full, Complete, and Correct Account of the Horrid Murder of the Poor Italian Boy Carlo Ferriar* (London: Dean and Munday 1831), 7, Wellcome Collection.
68 Waite, "Grave Robbing in New England," 284–85.
69 Rachel H. Mathis, Jill H. Watras, Jonathan M. Dort, "Grave Robbing in the North and South in Antebellum America," *American College of Surgeons* (2016): 16, https://www.facs.org/media/1x0f0byz/03_grave_robbing.pdf.
70 George Bergner, *The Legislative Record: Containing the Debates and Proceedings of the Pennsylvania Legislature, for The Session of 1863* (Harrisburg: Telegraph Steam Book and Job Office, 1863), 437, HathiTrust.
71 Ibid., 616.
72 Ibid., 617.
73 Ibid., 615.
74 *Detroit Free Press* (Detroit, MI), December 31, 1875.
75 Bergner, *The Legislative Record*, 616.
76 Ibid., 619.
77 Ibid., 615.
78 Ibid., 437.
79 Ibid., 615.

80 Ibid., 615.
81 William S. Forbes, *History of the Anatomy Act of Pennsylvania* (Philadelphia: The Philadelphia Medical Publishing Company, 1898), 11–12, Jefferson Digital Commons.
82 Ibid., 9.
83 "The Murderer's Body," *The Philadelphia Inquirer* (Philadelphia, PA), December 29, 1869, ProQuest.
84 "Horrors of the Morgue," *Chicago Tribune* (Chicago, IL), August 22, 1873, Newspapers.com.
85 "'Body Snatchers' At Work," *The Times* (Philadelphia, PA), June 16, 1875.
86 "A Premature Resurrection," *The Times* (Philadelphia, PA), August 1, 1876.
87 Ibid.
88 Ibid.

Chapter 7: "Jefferson's Resurrection Keys": Body Snatching on Trial

1 Edward Warren, *The Life of John Warren, M.D.* (Boston: Noyes, Holmes, and Company, 1874), 233, Uniformed Services University Archives.
2 Wunsch, "Parceling the Picturesque: 'Rural' Cemeteries and Urban Context in Nineteenth-Century Philadelphia," 148.
3 Lori Wysong, "Cemeteries, Segregation, and the Funerals of Henry Jones," Hidden City, accessed October 19, 2020, https://hiddencityphila.org/2020/10/cemeteries-segregation-and-the-funerals-of-henry-jones/.
4 P. Frazer Smith, *Pennsylvania State Reports Vol. LXXXI Comprising Cases Adjudged in the Supreme Court of Pennsylvania* (Philadelphia: Kay & Brother, 1877), 238, 241.
5 Smith, *Pennsylvania State Reports*, 236.
6 Wysong, "Cemeteries, Segregation, and the Funerals of Henry Jones."
7 "The Cemetery Trustees," *The Philadelphia Press* (Philadelphia, PA), December 6, 1882.
8 "Precautions in Philadelphia Cemeteries," *The Jeffersonian Democrat* (Brookville, PA), December 11, 1878.
9 "Digging Up the Dead," *The Philadelphia Press* (Philadelphia, PA), December 5, 1882.
10 Steven J. Peitzman, "City of Medicine," The Encyclopedia of Greater Philadelphia, accessed January 22, 2025, https://philadelphiaencyclopedia.org/essays/anatomy-and-anatomy-education/.
11 "The Body-Stealers' Plot," *The Philadelphia Press* (Philadelphia, PA), December 5, 1882.
12 Ibid.
13 "Mayer's Admission," *The Philadelphia Press* (Philadelphia, PA), December 5, 1882.
14 "Last Night's Capture," *The Philadelphia Press* (Philadelphia, PA), December 5, 1882.
15 Ibid.
16 Ibid.

17 George Wharton Pepper and William Draper Lewis, *A Digest of the Laws of Pennsylvania From 1700 To 1984* (Philadelphia: T. & J. W. Johnson & Co., 1896), 516–17.
18 "Digging Up Coffins," *The Philadelphia Inquirer* (Philadelphia, PA), December 7, 1882.
19 "The Press' Capture," *The Philadelphia Press* (Philadelphia, PA), December 5, 1882.
20 "Secrets of a Dissecting Room," *The Times* (New Bloomfield, PA), March 2, 1880.
21 Roger Lane, *Roots of Violence in Black Philadelphia, 1860–1900* (Cambridge: Harvard University Press, 1986), 85–86.
22 Thomas H. Keels, *Wicked Philadelphia: Sin In The City of Brotherly Love* (Charleston: The History Press, 2010), 52.
23 Lane, *The Roots of Violence in Black Philadelphia*, 64.
24 Leland M. Williamson, Richard A. Foley, Henry H. Colclazer, Louis N. Megargee, Jay H. Mowbray, William R. Antisdel, *Prominent and Progressive Pennsylvanians of the Nineteenth Century: Volume 1* (Philadelphia: The Record Publishing Company, 1898), 307, Internet Archive; *Lippincott's Monthly Magazine. A Popular Journal of General Literature, Science, and Politics* Vol. LII—July to December 1893 (Philadelphia: J. B. Lippincott Company, 1893), 734.
25 "The Press' Capture," *The Philadelphia Press* (Philadelphia, PA), December 5, 1882.
26 "The Bodies in the Morgue," *The Philadelphia Press* (Philadelphia, PA), December 6, 1882.
27 "Indignation Meetings," *The Philadelphia Press* (Philadelphia, PA), December 6, 1882.
28 "Scenes in the Cemetery," *The Philadelphia Press* (Philadelphia, PA), December 6, 1882.
29 "Trustee Burton at Bay," *The Times* (Philadelphia, PA), December 8, 1882.
30 *The Christian Recorder* (Philadelphia, PA), June 29, 1867, and February 1, 1868.
31 "The Ghouls Denounced," *The Philadelphia Press* (Philadelphia, PA), December 8, 1882.
32 Ibid.
33 *The Christian Recorder* (Philadelphia, PA), December 14, 1882, and December 7, 1882.
34 "Digging Up Coffins," *The Philadelphia Inquirer* (Philadelphia, PA), December 7, 1882.
35 "A Tale of Horror," *The Harrisburg Daily* (Harrisburg, PA), December 9, 1882.
36 *The Germantown Telegraph* (Philadelphia, PA), March 21, 1883.
37 Guerrasio, "Dissecting the Pennsylvania Anatomy Act," 35.
38 "Guarding the Ghouls," *The Philadelphia Press* (Philadelphia, PA), December 6, 1882; "The Body-Stealers' Plot," *The Philadelphia Press* (Philadelphia, PA), December 5, 1882.
39 "Guarding the Ghouls," *The Philadelphia Press* (Philadelphia, PA), December 6, 1882.
40 "Jefferson's Resurrection Keys," *The Philadelphia Press* (Philadelphia, PA), December 6, 1882.

41 "An Hour with Dr. Forbes," *The Philadelphia Press* (Philadelphia, PA), December 8, 1882.
42 Ibid.
43 "The Scene at Jefferson College," *The Philadelphia Press* (Philadelphia, PA), December 6, 1882.
44 "Body-Snatchers Held," *The Philadelphia Inquirer* (Philadelphia, PA), December 9, 1882.
45 "Guarding the Graves," *The Philadelphia Press* (Philadelphia, PA), December 13, 1882.
46 "The Ghouls," *The Philadelphia Inquirer* (Philadelphia, PA), December 16, 1882.
47 James R. Wright, Jr., "The Pennsylvania Anatomy Act of 1883: Weighing the Roles of Professor William Smith Forbes and Senator William James McKnight," *Journal of the History of Medicine and Allied Sciences*, 71, no. 4 (2016).
48 Frederick B. Wagner, Jr., M.D., J. Woodrow Savacool, M.D., eds., *Legend and Lore: Jefferson Medical College* (William T. Cooke Publishing, Inc., Devon, PA, 2009), 203, Jefferson Digital Commons, https://jdc.jefferson.edu/savacool/7.
49 McKnight, *A Pioneer Outline History of Northwestern Pennsylvania*, 300.
50 "Dead For The Doctors," *The Christian Recorder* (Philadelphia, PA), December 28, 1882.
51 Forbes, *History of the Anatomy Act*, 17.
52 Forbes, *History of the Anatomy Act*, 17.
53 McKnight, *A Pioneer Outline History of Northwestern Pennsylvania*, 302.
54 Forbes, *History of the Anatomy Act*, 23.
55 Keels, *Wicked Philadelphia*, 58.
56 Forbes, *History of the Anatomy Act*, 24.
57 Ibid., 24.
58 McKnight, *A Pioneer Outline History of Northwestern Pennsylvania*, 308.
59 "The Defect of the Anatomy Act," *The Times* (Philadelphia, PA), December 27, 1882.
60 "Dr. Forbes on Trial," *The Philadelphia Press* (Philadelphia, PA), March 13, 1883.
61 "The Defect of the Anatomy Act," *The Times* (Philadelphia, PA), December 27, 1882; "Grave-Robbing and the Remedy," *The Times* (Philadelphia, PA), March 18, 1883.
62 Sievers, *The Harrison Horror*, 13.
63 "Dr. Forbes on Trial," *The Philadelphia Press* (Philadelphia, PA), March 13, 1883.
64 "In the Jury's Hands," *The Philadelphia Press* (Philadelphia, PA), March 17, 1883.
65 "The Forbes Jury Out," *The Times* (Philadelphia, PA), March 17, 1883.
66 "Dr. Forbes' Trial," *The Philadelphia Inquirer* (Philadelphia, PA), March 15, 1883.
67 "The Hearing," *The Philadelphia Press* (Philadelphia, PA), December 9, 1882.
68 "Secrets of the Dissecting-Room," *The Philadelphia Press* (Philadelphia, PA), December 5, 1882.
69 Wright, "The Pennsylvania Anatomy Act of 1883," 436.

70 "Our Philadelphia Letter," *Washington Bee* (Washington, D.C.), March 24, 1883.
71 "Sequel to a Grave Robbery," *The Philadelphia Record* (Philadelphia, PA), May 10, 1886.
72 Lawrence, *History of the Philadelphia Almshouses and Hospitals*, 317.
73 *The College and Clinical Record* V, no. 4 (April 1, 1884): 100, Jefferson Digital Commons.
74 "Stolen From His Grave," *Cincinnati Enquirer* (Cincinnati, OH), July 17, 1884, ProQuest.
75 "The May Ghouls," *The Philadelphia Inquirer* (Philadelphia, PA), August 8, 1884.
76 Guerrasio, "Dissecting the Pennsylvania Anatomy Act."
77 *American Medicine*, American-Medicine Publishing Company IX, no. 8 (February 25, 1905).
78 Thomas H. Keels, *Philadelphia Graveyards and Cemeteries* (Charleston: Arcadia Publishing, 2003), 84; Wysong, "Cemeteries, Segregation, and the Funerals of Henry Jones."
79 Erin McLeary, "The Curious Case Of Body Snatching At Lebanon Cemetery," Hidden City, accessed December 1, 2024, https://hiddencityphila.org/2015/04/the-curious-case-of-body-snatching-at-lebanon-cemetery/#:~:text=The%20Press%20alleged%20that%20Lebanon,had%20been%20taken%20for%20dissection.
80 "Ghoul is Murdered," *The Hanford Sentinel* (Hanford, CA), December 31, 1903.
81 "Louis N. Megargee Has Passed Away," *The Philadelphia Inquirer* (Philadelphia, PA), December 27, 1905, ProQuest.
82 "Historic Brookville Sees New State Historical Marker," *Courier Express* (DuBois, PA), November 1, 2018, http://www.thecourierexpress.com/historic-brookville-sees-new-state-historical-marker/article_ca238335-8b4e-5b06-b7c5-37533eccea37.html.
83 Wright, "The Pennsylvania Anatomy Act of 1883," 433.
84 "Workmen Find Tidal Springs In Excavation For Hospital," *The Philadelphia Inquirer* (Philadelphia, PA), July 22, 1903, ProQuest.

Afterword: The Legacy of Body Snatching

1 "The Race to Save Benjamin Franklin's Cracked Gravestone," Mental Floss, accessed December 1, 2024, https://www.mentalfloss.com/article/501106/race-save-benjamin-franklins-cracked-gravestone.
2 "Arch Street Project Examines Life and Death in Colonial Philadelphia," Hidden City, accessed December 1, 2024, https://hiddencityphila.org/2022/07/arch-street-project-examines-life-and-death-in-colonial-philadelphia/.
3 "Playing on Hallowed Ground: Hidden Cemeteries and the Modern City," Hidden City, accessed December 1, 2024, https://hiddencityphila.org/2020/02/playing-on-hallowed-ground-hidden-cemeteries-and-the-modern-city/.

4 "The Resurrectionists," *Frank Leslie's Illustrated Newspaper* (New York City, NY), January 6, 1866, History Commons.
5 "In Philadelphia, finding dignity for bodies left unclaimed," WHYY, accessed December 1, 2024, https://whyy.org/segments/in-philadelphia-finding-dignity-for-bodies-left-unclaimed/.
6 Ibid.
7 "Three decades ago, Philly's medical examiner sent 26 human brains to a Penn professor without consent," Billy Penn, accessed December 1, 2024, https://billypenn.com/2021/07/31/philadelphia-brains-medical-examiner-university-pennsylvania-lawsuit-move-remains/.
8 "United States of America vs. CEDRIC LODGE, KATRINA MACLEAN, JOSHUA TAYLOR and DENISE LODGE," United States District Court Middle District of Pennsylvania, accessed December 1, 2024, 9, https://media.wbur.org/wp/2023/06/morgue-indictment.pdf.
9 Ally Jarmanning, "Harvard, The Human Remains Trade, and Collectors Who Fuel the Market," WBUR, accessed December 1, 2024, https://www.wbur.org/news/2024/06/13/harvard-medical-anatomy-human-remains-network.
10 Paul Wolff Mitchell, "Black Philadelphians in the Samuel George Morton Cranial Collection," Penn Program On Race, Science & Society, last modified February 15, 2021, https://prss.sas.upenn.edu/projects/penn-medicines-role/black-philadelphians-samuel-george-morton-cranial-collection.
11 "Penn Museum will no longer display exposed human remains," WHYY, accessed December 1, 2024, https://whyy.org/articles/penn-museum-no-longer-display-exposed-human-remains/.
12 "Mütter Museum launches public engagement program over the future of its collection," WHYY, accessed December 1, 2024, https://whyy.org/articles/mutter-museum-public-engagement-program-collection-future/#:~:text=According%20to%20the%20museum%2C%20it,was%20acquired%20through%20informed%20consent.

Appendix

1 Forbes, *History of the Anatomy Act*, 23–25.

Selected Bibliography

Primary Sources

Agnew, David Hayes, Alfred Stille, Lewis P. Bush, Charles K. Mills, and Roland G. Curtin. *History and Reminiscences of the Philadelphia Almshouse and Philadelphia Hospital.* Philadelphia, PA: Detre & Blackburn, 1890, HathiTrust.

Agnew, David Hayes. "The Medical History of the Philadelphia Almshouse." In *History of Blockley: A History of the Philadelphia General Hospital from Its Inception, 1731–1928*, edited by John Welsh Croskey. Philadelphia, PA: F. A. Davis Company, 1929.

Bailey, James Blake. *The Diary of a Resurrectionist 1811–1812.* London, UK: Swan Sonnenschein & Co., 1896, Project Gutenberg.

Baker, Frank. "A History of Bodysnatching." In *Washington Medical Annals (Bimonthly) Journal of the Medical Society of the District of Columbia Vol. XV, 1916.* City of Washington: Beresford, Printer, 1916, Internet Archive.

Bliss, Arthur Ames. *Blockley Days: Memories and Impressions of a Resident Physician 1883–1884.* Springfield, MA: Springfield Printing & Binding Co., 1916.

Dixon, Edward H. "Scenes in a Medical Student's Life—Resurrectionizing." *Scalpel: An Entirely Original Quarterly Expositor of the Laws of Health, and Abuses of Medicine and Domestic Life* 7 (1855), Gale.

Forbes, William S. *History of the Anatomy Act of Pennsylvania.* Philadelphia, PA: The Philadelphia Medical Publishing Company, 1898, Jefferson Digital Commons.

Hartwell, Edward Mussey. "The Hindrances to Anatomical Study in the United States, Including a Special Record of the Struggles of Our Early Anatomical Teachers." In *Annals of Anatomy and Surgery: The Journal of the Anatomical and Surgical Society*, edited by Lewis S. Pilcher and George R. Fowler. Brooklyn: 1881, HathiTrust.

Juettner, Otto. *Daniel Drake and His Followers: Historical and Biographical Sketches.* Cincinnati, OH: Harvey Publishing Company, 1909, HathiTrust.

Lawrence, Charles. *History of the Philadelphia Almshouses and Hospitals.* Self-published, 1905.

McKnight, W. J. *A Pioneer Outline History of Northwestern Pennsylvania.* Philadelphia, PA: J. B. Lippincott Company, 1905.

Warren, Edward. *The Life of John Collins Warren, M.D. Compiled Chiefly from His Autobiography and Journals in Two Volumes. Vol. I.* Boston, MA: Ticknor and Fields, 1860, Google Books.

Watson, John Fanning. *Annals of Philadelphia and Pennsylvania, In the Olden Time Vol. I.* Self-published, 1884, Internet Archive.

Watson, John Fanning. *Annals of Philadelphia and Pennsylvania, In the Olden Time Vol. II.* Self-published, 1850, Internet Archive.

Webster, James. *Facts Concerning Anatomical Instruction in Philadelphia.* Philadelphia, PA: 1832, Wellcome Collection.

Secondary Sources

Atlas Obscura. "Victorian 'Coffin Torpedoes' Blasted Would-Be Body Snatchers." Accessed April 28, 2024. https://www.atlasobscura.com/articles/coffin-torpedos.

Baatz, Simon. "'A Very Diffused Disposition': Dissecting Schools in Philadelphia, 1823–1825." *The Pennsylvania Magazine of History and Biography* 108, no. 2 (1984).

Berry, Daina Ramey. *The Price for Their Pound of Flesh: The Value of the Enslaved, from Womb to Grave, in the Building of a Nation.* Boston, MA: Beacon Press, 2017.

Breeden, James O. "Body Snatchers and Anatomy Professors: Medical Education in Nineteenth-Century Virginia." *The Virginia Magazine of History and Biography* 83, no. 3 (July 1975), JSTOR.

Corner, Betsy Copping. *William Shippen, Jr., Pioneer in American Medical Education.* Philadelphia: American Philosophical Society, 1951, HathiTrust.

Diseroad, Ann F. "Were they to keep the dead in…or the living out? CAGES ON GRAVES EXPLAINED A Wee Bit of Olde Scotland Right Here in Columbia County." Columbia County Historical & Genealogical Society Newsletter Article. Accessed April 27, 2024, https://colcohist-gensoc.org/wp-content/uploads/Cages%20on%20Graves%20Explained.pdf.

Edwards, Linden F. *Cincinnati's "Old Cunny": A Notorious Purveyor of Human Flesh.* Public Library of Fort Wayne and Allen County, 1955, Project Gutenberg.

Gerstner, Patsy. "A Note on Body Snatching in the United States." *The Bulletin of the Cleveland Medical Library* 18, no. 7 (July 1971).

Guerrasio, Venetia M. "Dissecting the Pennsylvania Anatomy Act: Laws, Bodies, and Science, 1880–1960." PhD diss., University of New Hampshire, Durham, 2007. University of New Hampshire Scholars Repository (376).

Harra, Todd. *Last Rites: The Evolution of the American Funeral.* Boulder, CO: Sounds True, 2022.

Kaufman, Martin and Hanawalt, Leslie L. "Body Snatching in the Midwest." *Michigan History Magazine* 55, no. 1 (1971).

Lennox, Suzie. *Bodysnatchers: Digging Up the Untold Stories of Britain's Resurrection Men.* Yorkshire, UK: Pen & Sword History, 2016.

Moore, Wendy. *The Knife Man: Blood, Body Snatching, and the Birth of Modern Surgery.* New York: Broadway Books, 2005.

Prothero, Stephen. *Purified by Fire: A History of Cremation in America.* Berkeley, CA: University of California Press, 2001.

Richardson, Ruth. *Death, Dissection and the Destitute.* Chicago, IL: The University of Chicago Press, 2000.

Sappol, Michael. *A Traffic of Dead Bodies: Anatomy and Embodied Social Identity in Nineteenth-Century America.* Princeton, NJ: Princeton University Press, 2002.

Shultz, Suzanne M. *Body Snatching: The Robbing of Graves for the Education of Physicians in Early Nineteenth Century America.* Jefferson: McFarland & Company, 1992.

Sievers, Harry J. *The Harrison Horror.* Fort Wayne: Public Library of Fort Wayne and Allen County, 1956, HathiTrust.

Sozinsky, T. S. "Grave-Robbing and Dissection." *The Penn Monthly* 10 (January–December 1879), HathiTrust.

Wilf, Steven Robert. "Anatomy and Punishment in Late Eighteenth-Century New York." *Journal of Social History* 22, no. 3 (spring 1989), JSTOR.

Waite, Dr. Frederick C. "Grave Robbing in New England." *Bulletin of the Medical Library Association* 33, no. 3 (July 1945).

Wright Jr., James R. "The Pennsylvania Anatomy Act of 1883: Weighing the Roles of Professor William Smith Forbes and Senator William James McKnight." *Journal of the History of Medicine and Allied Sciences* 71, no. 4 (2016).

Index